NETWORK EPIDEMIOLOGY

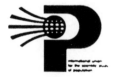

The International Union for the Scientific Study of Population Problems was set up in 1928, with Dr Raymond Pearl as President. At that time the Union's main purpose was to promote international scientific co-operation to study the various aspects of population problems, through national committees and through its members themselves. In 1947 the International Union for the Scientific Study of Population (IUSSP) was reconstituted into its present form.
   It expanded its activities to:

- stimulate research on population
- develop interest in demographic matters among governments, national and international organizations, scientific bodies, and the general public
- foster relations between people involved in population studies
- disseminate scientific knowledge on population.

The principal ways through which the IUSSP currently achieves its aims are:

- organization of worldwide or regional conferences
- operations of Scientific Committees under the auspices of the Council
- organization of training courses
- publication of conference proceedings and committee reports.

Demography can be defined by its field of study and its analytical methods. Accordingly, it can be regarded as the scientific study of human populations primarily with respect to their size, their structure, and their development. For reasons which are related to the history of the discipline, the demographic method is essentially inductive: progress in knowledge results from the improvement of observation, the sophistication of measurement methods, and the search for regularities and stable factors leading to the formulation of explanatory models. In conclusion, the three objectives of demographic analysis are to describe, measure, and analyse.

International Studies in Demography is the outcome of an agreement concluded by the IUSSP and the Oxford University Press. The joint series reflects the broad range of the Union's activities; it is based on the seminars organized by the Union and important international meetings in the field of population and development. The Editorial Board of the series is comprised of:

Network Epidemiology: A Handbook for Survey Design and Data Collection

Edited by

MARTINA MORRIS

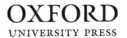

OXFORD
UNIVERSITY PRESS

This book has been printed digitally and produced in a standard specification
in order to ensure its continuing availability

OXFORD
UNIVERSITY PRESS

Great Clarendon Street, Oxford OX2 6DP

Oxford University Press is a department of the University of Oxford.
It furthers the University's objective of excellence in research, scholarship,
and education by publishing worldwide in

Oxford New York

Auckland Cape Town Dar es Salaam Hong Kong Karachi
Kuala Lumpur Madrid Melbourne Mexico City Nairobi
New Delhi Shanghai Taipei Toronto
With offices in
Argentina Austria Brazil Chile Czech Republic France Greece
Guatemala Hungary Italy Japan South Korea Poland Portugal
Singapore Switzerland Thailand Turkey Ukraine Vietnam

Oxford is a registered trade mark of Oxford University Press
in the UK and in certain other countries

Published in the United States
by Oxford University Press Inc., New York

© IUSSP, 2004

The moral rights of the author have been asserted

Database right Oxford University Press (maker)

Reprinted 2007

ISBN 978-0-19-926901-3

Contents

PART III. COMPLETE NETWORK DESIGNS

Acknowledgments

This book would not have been possible without many years of patient support and encouragement from the IUSSP and the United States National Institutes of Health (NIH). Let me start by thanking the original members of the IUSSP Working Group on AIDS – Kofi Awusabo-Asare, Ties Boerma, Michel Carael, Hans Hansen, Anchalee Singhanetra-Renard, and our fearless leader Basia Zaba – for supporting the original idea of a conference organized around a set of research teams that led to this volume. Anchalee was the local organizer of that conference, which was hosted by the Regional Center for Sustainable Development at Chiang-Mai University, and she did a wounderful job of linking international visitors to local Thai scholars and students. We were lucky to have Renee Latour as the IUSSP coordinator for the conference – anything we needed, it was done; she made things seem so easy. The Population Research Institute at Penn State University provided superb logistical support for the project website. The NIH provided support for my work on the conference and this subsequent volume through several grants over the years (R29 HD34957, R01 DA12831, and R01 HD41877). I would particularly like to thank the staff at the Demographic and Behavioral Science Branch of NICHD, especially my project officer, Susan Newcomer, who attended the conference and has supported this work from the beginning. Cynthia Pearson, Sarah Gelfand, and Claire Lev helped with the editorial tasks here at the University of Washington, and their work has made this a much more coherent and well-organized volume. Finally, I would like to thank the editorial staff at OUP – they have been a delight to work with.

List of Contributors

Aral, Sevgi O., Associate Director for Science, Division of STD Prevention, Centers for Disease Control & Prevention, MS E02, 1600 Clifton Road, Atlanta, GA 30333, USA, Tel: +1 404 639 8259, Fax: +1 404 639 8608, soal@cdc.gov

Baldwin, Juliet, Co-Director, Department of Health, Physical Education, Exercise Science, and Nutrition, Northern Arizona University, PO Box 15095, Flagstaff, AZ 86011-5095 USA, Tel: +1 520-523-8261, Fax: 520-523-4315, Julie.Baldwin@nau.edu

Bearman, Peter S., Institute for Social and Economic Theory and Research, Columbia University, 814 SIPA Building, Columbia University, New York, NY 10027, Tel: (212) 854-3094, Fax: (212) 854-8925, psb17@columbia.edu

Caraël, Michael, UNAIDS, 20 Avenue Appia, CH-1211 Geneva 27, Switzerland, Tel: +41 22 791 4611, Fax: +41 22 791 4746

Darrow, William W., Florida International University, Miami, USA

Entwisle, Barbara, Professor Department of Sociology and Director, Carolina Population Center, University of North Carolina at Chapel Hill, CB# 8120, 123 West Franklin Street, Chapel Hill, NC 27516, USA, Tel: 919-966-1710, Fax: 919-966-6638, entwisle@unc.edu

Faust, Katherine, Associate Professor of Sociology, University of California, Irvine, Irvine, CA 92697-5100, USA, Tel: 949-824-9383, Fax: 949-824-4717, kfaust@uci.edu

Foxman, Betsy, Professor of Epidemiology, Director, Center for Molecular and Clinical Epidemiology of Infectious Diseases, University of Michigan School of Public Health Department of Epidemiology, 109 Observatory Street, Ann Arbor, MI 48109-2020 USA, Tel: (734) 764-5487, Fax: (734) 764-3192, bfoxman@umich.edu

Garnett, Geoff, Professor of Microparasite Epidemiology, Department of Infectious Disease Epidemiology, Imperial College, St Mary's Campus, London SW7 2AZ, UK, Tel: 020 759 43283, Fax: 020 7262 3495, g.garnett@imperial.ac.uk

Glynn, Judith R., Infectious Disease Epidemiology Unit, London School of Hygiene and Tropical Medicine, Keppel St, London WC1E 7HT, UK

Golden, Matthew, Acting Instructor, Center for AIDS and STD / Allergy and Infectious Diseases, and Medical Director, Public Health—Seattle & King County STD Clinic, Harborview Medical Center, Box 359931, 325 Ninth Avenue, Seattle, WA 98104-2499, USA, Tel: +1 206-731-6829; Fax: +1 206-731-3693, golden@u.washington.edu

Gorbach, Pamina M., Assistant Professor, in Residence, Department of Epidemiology, Box 951772, Los Angeles, CA 90095-1772, USA, Tel: +1 310-267-2805, Fax: +1 310-825-8440, pgorbach@ucla.edu

Holmes, King K., Director, Center for AIDS and STD Head, Infectious Diseases, Allergy & Infectious Diseases, Harborview Medical Center, Box 359931, 325 Ninth Avenue, Seattle, WA 98104-2499, USA, Tel: +1 206-731-3620, Fax: +1 206-731-3694, worthy@u.washington.edu

Hughes, James P., Associate Professor, Biostatistics, Harborview Medical Center, Box 359931, 325 Ninth Avenue Seattle, WA 98104-2499, USA, Tel: +1 206-731-3633, +1 206-616-2721, jphughes@u.washington.edu

Jampaklay, Aree, Lecturer, Institute for Population and Social Research, Mahidol University, Phutthamonthon, Nakhorn Pathom, 73170 Thailand, Tel 662-441-9667 ext. 206, Fax: 662-441-9333, praun@mahidol.ac.th or jampakla@email.unc.edu

Klovdahl, Alden S., The Australian National University, Canberra, Australia

Lagarde, Emmanuel, INSERM U88/IFR 69, 14 rue du Val d'Osne, 94410 Saint Maurice, France, Tel: 33 1 45 18 38 58, Fax: 33 1 45 18 38 89, emmanuel.lagarde@st-maurice.inserm.fr

Laumann, Edward O., George Herbert Mead Distinguished Service Professor of Sociology and the College, Department of Sociology, University of Chicago, 5848 S. University Avenue, Chicago, IL 60637, Tel: (773) 702-4610, Fax: (773) 702-4607, e-laumann@uchicago.edu

Long, David, Independent Investigator

Mahay, Jenna, NIA Post-doctoral Fellow, Center on Demography and Economics of Aging, University of Chicago, 1155 East 60th South, Chicago, IL 60637, Tel: (773) 256-6338, Fax: (773) 245-6313, j-mahay@uchicago.edu

Manhart, Lisa E., Post-doctoral Fellow, Center for AIDS and STD / Allergy and Infectious Diseases, Harborview Medical Center, Box 359931, 325 Ninth Avenue, Seattle, WA 98104-2499, USA, Tel: +1 206-731-3646; Fax: +1 206-731-3693, lmanhart@u.washington.edu

Maxwell, Carol, Independent Investigator

Moody, James, Associate Professor, Department of Sociology, 372 Bricker Hall, 190 North Oval Mall, The Ohio State University, Columbus, OH 43215, USA, Tel: (614) 292-1722, Fax: 614-292-6687, moody.77@osu.edu

Morison, Linda, Infectious Disease Epidemiology Unit, London School of Hygiene and Tropical Medicine, Keppel St, London WC1E 7HT, UK

Morris, Martina, Center for Studies of Demography and Ecology, University of Washington, Box 353412 Seattle, WA 98195-3412, morrism@u.washington.edu

Muth, John B., El Paso County Department of Health & Environment, Colorado Springs, USA

Muth, Stephen Q., El Paso County Department of Health & Environment, Colorado Springs, USA

Pach, Albert, Independent Investigator

Paik, Anthony, Assistant Professor, Department of Sociology, University of Iowa, 140 Seashore Hall West, Iowa City, IA 52242, Tel: (319) 335-2493, Fax: (319) 335-2509, anthony-paik@uiowa.edu

Podhisita, Chai, Institute for Population and Social Research, Mahidol Univ., Salaya, Nakhon Pathom, 73170 Thailand. Phone: (66)-2-441-0201-4, 441-9518-9 Ext. 276 Fax: (66)-2-441-9333, prcps@mahidol.ac.th

Potterat, John J., Former Director, STD/HIV Programs, El Paso County Department of Health and Environment, 301 South Union Blvd, Colorado Springs, CO 80910-3123, USA; and Independent Consultant, 301 South Union Blvd, Colorado Springs, CO 80910, Tel: (719) 632-3120, Fax: +1 719 637 3032, jjpotterat@earthlink.net

Prasartkul, Pramote, Professor, Institute for Population and Social Research, Mahidol University, Phutthamonthon, Nakhorn Pathom, 73170 Thailand, Tel: 662-441-0201-4 ext. 214, Fax: 662-441-9333, prpps@mahidol.ac.th

Rindfuss, Ronald R., Professor, Department of Sociology and Carolina Population Center, University of North Carolina at Chapel Hill, CB# 8120, 123 West Franklin Street, Chapel Hill, NC 27516, USA, Tel: 919-966-7779, Fax: 919-966-6638, ron_rindfuss@unc.edu

Rothenberg, Richard B., Department of Family and Preventive Medicine, Emory University School of Medicine, 69 Jesse Hill Jr Drive, SE, Atlanta, GA 30303, Tel: 404 616 5606, Fax: 404 616 6847, Pager: 404 866 8575, rrothen@emory.edu

Sawangdee, Yothin, Assistant Professor, Institute for Population and Social Research, Mahidol University, Phutthamonthon, Nakhorn Pathom, 73170 Thailand, Tel: 662-441-0201-4 ext. 303, Fax: 662-441-9333, prysw@mahidol.ac.th

Sewankambo, Nelson K., M.D. Uganda National Council of Science and Technology, Makerere Medical School P.O. Box 7072 Kampala, Uganda Phone: (256-41) 558731/557505. sewankam@infocom.co.ug.

Sterk, Claire, Department of Behavioral Sciences and Health Education, Rollins School of Public Health, Emory University, Atlanta, GA

Stoner, Bradley P., Associate Professor of Medicine, Chief of STD Services, St Louis County Department of Health, Department of Anthropology, Washington University, 1 Brookings Drive, Campus Box 1114, St Louis 63130, USA, Tel: (314) 935-5673, Fax: (314) 935-8535, bstoner@artsci.wustl.edu

Stovel, Katherine, Assistant Professor, Sociology, Box 353340, University of Washington, Seattle, WA 98195, USA, Tel: +1 206-616-3820, Fax: +1 206-543-2516, stovel@u.washington.edu

Thalji, Lisa, Staff Member, RTI, PO Box 12194, Research Triangle Park, NC 27709-2194; Tel: +1 919-485-2666.

Trotter, Robert Talbot II, Regents' Professor, Department of Anthropology, PO Box 15200, Flagstaff, AZ 86011, USA, Tel: +1 928/523-4521, Fax: +1 928/523-9135, Robert.Trotter@nau.edu

Wawer, Maria, M.D., M.H., S.c., Professor of Clinical Population & Family Health, Columbia University School of Public Health, 60 HAVEN AVE B-2, New York, NY 10032. Tel: +1 212-304-5278, Fax: +1 212-304-5272, mjw4@columbia.edu

Woodhouse, Donald E., El Paso County Department of Health & Environment, Colorado Springs, USA

Youm, Yoosik, Assistant Professor, Department of Sociology, University of Illinois at Chicago, 1007 West Harrison (M/C 312), Chicago, IL 60607, Tel: (312) 996-5935, Fax: (312) 996-5104, yoosik@uic.edu

List of Figures

List of Tables

Editor's Introduction

MARTINA MORRIS

This book is the outcome of a conference on "Partnerships and the Spread of HIV and Other Infections" sponsored by the International Union for the Scientific Study of Population (IUSSP) in Chiang Mai, Thailand in February 2000. The purpose of the conference was to synthesize a decade's worth of new empirical research that has used network analytic methods to understand the population dynamics of HIV, and make it accessible to the larger research community. Interest in social network analysis has grown rapidly among applied researchers in the population sciences—starting with epidemiologists working on the HIV/AIDS epidemic in the mid 1980s and moving quickly into many other areas in demography. Methods for network analysis have been under development during the past 50 years (Wasserman and Faust 1994), and the theory is rooted in the classic works of anthropology (e.g. Levi-Strauss 1969), but it is only in the last decade or so that this work is beginning to find a broader audience among applied researchers. A good example is the academic and popular attention now given to "small world" diffusion models (Watts 1999; Barabasi 2002; Watts 2003), the variations on the "six degrees of separation" game (see, e.g. www.cs.virginia.edu/oracle), and the range of computer viruses that regularly make their way into our email inboxes. As a result of this new attention, the pace of progress in the field of network analysis has increased, and the volume and range of new work coming out in this area is now quite remarkable.

Conducting empirical studies of networks, however, remains quite a challenge. It requires many changes in research design, and there is currently no source in the published literature that an interested researcher could turn to for a systematic introduction to these issues. The Chiang Mai conference was set up to produce such a handbook, and this is the result. The conference was explicitly organized to ensure that the presentations covered the range of issues relevant for network research: from the impact it has on data collection instruments and sampling, to the changes it requires in statistical methodology, and finally, to what we have learned from network studies in perhaps the most active research context to use these tools: the epidemic spread of HIV.

The central presentations at the conference were made by six research teams with long-standing empirical projects involving network survey research. These are not the only projects that have been undertaken in the past 10 years, but they include some of the earliest and most ambitious.[1] They were selected to provide a good introduction to the range of survey strategies available, and to highlight the way that partnership networks span physical space, social space, and time. The projects were located in many regions of the world: multiple locations in the United States, rural and urban areas in Thailand, and several countries in sub-Saharan Africa. Each session of the

---

[1] An important pioneer not included here is the "Bushwick Study" of injection drug users in New York City (Friedman et al. 1997).

conference focused on a single project, and three or four members of the project team made a joint presentation. The sessions were long (2 h) and were set sequentially rather than concurrently to maximize the potential interactions among research teams with different methods. Our intention was to broaden the usual focus of discussion to include the actual conduct of the research, as well as the findings.

Network analysis is still a young field. Given the range of different network sampling strategies, the absence of training in network methods in most disciplines, and the scarcity of empirical projects to collect network data, much research methodology is still learned and invented on the fly. The primary aim of the conference, and this subsequent volume, is to record what has been learned by the teams here. The result is substantially more than a random list of techniques and options, but also somewhat less than a simple recipe for doing empirical network research. There remain many unsolved challenges in this field, so it is a good time to consolidate what has been learned before moving on.

NETWORKS AND HIV

It is not coincidental that most of the projects presented in this volume focus on the global epidemic of HIV: the network perspective has challenged the way we approach HIV prevention. The influence goes both ways, though, as HIV has also challenged the way we approach network research. Over the past 15 years, the interaction between the practical need for policies to prevent the spread of HIV, and the basic social science research needed to address this need has been remarkably fruitful for both sides. We now understand much more about the population dynamics of infectious disease, and we also have developed network survey and analytic methodologies to a point where they are accessible to a wider range of researchers. The issues that have driven this progress are worth describing in brief.

On the one hand, networks offer us a more comprehensive way of thinking about individual behavior and its consequences for HIV. Unlike some health-related behavior (e.g. smoking and seat belts), behaviors that transmit HIV directly involve at least two people, and are also dependent on the other links either of these persons might have to others. This process cannot be studied or understood using the standard, individual-centered research paradigm. Moving away from this paradigm, however, has profound implications for the analytic framework, data collection, and intervention planning.

The analytic framework must move beyond the traditional focus on the individual to a relational analysis, in which the individual, the partnership, and the larger network can be integrated. This is a pretty radical shift in focus for most demographers and medical researchers. The theoretical framework that is needed takes us well away from what has become the standard approach to "behavioral research" that links individual attributes to individual outcomes. To the extent that an appropriate alternative framework has been developed, it is in the field of network research. So it is here that one should look for an orientation to the new principles: the analysis of position, groups, connectivity, and overall structure.

Data collection and statistical analysis need to be revised accordingly, making the partnership—rather than the individual—the primary sampling unit, and the cumulation rules of partnerships the primary analytic task. Again traditional research methodology comes up short. While we know a lot about sampling individuals, we know very little about sampling partnerships, and even less about sampling from networks. Capture–recapture techniques (Seber 1982; Fienberg 1992; Rubin et al. 1992; Hook and Regal 1995), adaptive sampling (Thompson and Seber 1996), and missing data methods (Little and Rubin 2002) are providing the first tools for network sampling (Frank and Snijders 1994; Thompson and Frank 2000). Once we solve the sampling problem, the defining property of such a sample is that the units are not independent. This violates the first assumption in virtually all the traditional statistical methods. Methods for analyzing dependent data are not unknown—spatial statistics (Besag 1974), time series (Shumway and Stoffer 2000), random graph models (Frank and Strauss 1986), and various multilevel models (Heck and Thomas 2000) provide a starting point—but the statistical tools needed to analyze networks have only begun to be developed (Wasserman and Pattison 1996; Snijders 2001; Hoff et al. 2002; Handcock 2003; Morris 2003).

The collection of network data also poses unique challenges with respect to issues of confidentiality and human subjects protection. The federal Office of Human Research Protections (OHRP) defines as "human subjects" anyone for whom a study collects individually identifiable, private information. The implications for social network research are profound, as the constraints imposed by the need to preserve confidentiality must be addressed at every stage of the research process. At this time, the implications of human subjects requirements for network data collection are the topic of much debate. Under the federal "Common Rule" informed consent must be obtained from any human subject of research, though this can be waived by an Institutional Review Board in certain limited circumstances. Depending on the design of a network study, this could mean that all identifiable partners nominated by enrolled study respondents would have to be found and consented before any information could be collected on them. A recent federal panel summarized the current understanding as follows:

In the course of participating in a research study, a human subject may provide information to investigators about other persons, such as a spouse, relative, friend, or social acquaintance. These other persons are referred to as "third parties." Over the last two years, questions have arisen in the research community about whether the Common Rule (regulations governing the protection of human subjects in Federally-funded research that are codified by the Department of Health and Humans Services at 45 CFR 46 Part A) applies to third parties in research and whether third parties are human subjects or can become human subjects during the course of research. The Common Rule does not specifically address third party information and its definition of "human subject" leaves some room for interpretation in this regard. (www.nih.gov/sigs/bioethics/nih_third_party_rec.html)

Confidentiality remains an issue in the management and analysis of network data. In contrast to more traditional social survey data, which is often publicly accessible and widely disseminated, network data often contain information that needs to be kept secure and protected from inappropriate disclosure. Researchers have struggled to find a balance between the conflicting norms of free access for scientific inquiry, and preserving the confidentiality of their research subjects. The challenge this poses is described in several of the chapters in this volume.

Finally, the network perspective changes the way we design effective HIV prevention strategies. First, it raises questions about targeting concepts such as "risk groups" and "risk behaviors." The inadequacy of these concepts has become clear as HIV-incidence surveys around the world reveal rising infection rates among groups that do not engage in individually risky behavior, for example, monogamous married women (Allen et al. 1991; Weniger et al. 1991; Guimaraes et al. 1995; Rodrigues et al. 1995). Similarly, a group of persons with extremely "risky" individual behavior may have little actual risk of HIV exposure if their partners are uninfected, and not linked to the rest of the partnership network. In short, it is not only individuals' behavior that defines their risk, it is their partner's behavior and (ultimately) their position in a network. Second, the risk of an epidemic at the population level is not simply a function of the individual behavior such as number of partners, it is also determined by the way the partnerships are connected. Serial monogamy in sexual partnerships creates a highly segmented network with no links between each pair of persons at any moment in time. Relax this constraint, allowing people to have multiple partners concurrently, and the network can become much more connected. The result is a massive increase in the spread of HIV, even if the mean number of partners per person does not change (Morris and Kretzschmar 1997). Finally, the fact that behavior occurs in the context of a partnership means that individual knowledge, attitudes, and beliefs do not affect behavior directly. Instead, the impact of these individual level variables is mediated by the relationship between the partners. A young woman who knows that condoms help prevent the sexual spread of HIV may be unable to convince her male partner to use one. It is not her knowledge that is deficient, it is her control over joint behavior.

Networks thus determine the level of individual exposure, the population dynamics of spread, and the interactional context that constrains behavioral change. Taking this seriously represents a paradigm shift in the study of HIV and other infectious diseases.

HIV AND NETWORK ANALYSIS

Not all of the influence has been from network analysis to HIV research. In fact, it would be hard to overestimate the reverse impact that HIV has had on the field of network analysis. For years, the methods developed in the field of network analysis required a census of the network: that is, complete data on every node and every link in the population of interest. While this has been an important starting point for establishing the kinds of questions a network approach can raise and answer, such data rarely become available in practice. As a result, the field of network analysis became fairly insular. A few well-known data sets, like the Sampson Monastery data, circulated around, analyzed, and reanalyzed as new methods were tested and compared to old. And in the absence of real and important data, the field became known for somewhat arcane mathematical developments rather than practical applications. The pace of progress was slow and comfortable.

The challenge of HIV, and the resources that have been focused on the basic science needed to contain the epidemic, changed all of this. As practitioners in public health came to recognize that we need to understand networks in order to prevent the spread of HIV, the world beat a path to network analysts' door. The analytic elegance of the complete network approach came face to face with the pressing need for a practical way to measure and analyze networks in different communities around the world. This created enormous pressure to develop more feasible alternatives for empirical research. The result has been a remarkable progress on mapping out the range of methods that can be used when some kind of sample is taken from the network. Local or "egocentric" network methods, long considered a poor, uninteresting cousin to complete network methods, became a key area for research. Local network methods rely on a simple random sample of respondents, who are then asked to describe their partners (their "local network"). In addition, the snowball sampling schemes used by public health contact tracers began to produce rich but complicated data which begged for analysis.

For the first time, data and important policy needs began to drive the development of network methodology. The result has been the emergence of a much larger and more interdisciplinary research community, and the development of a flexible set of research strategies that can be used in many different contexts.

The chapters in this book bear witness to the progress that has been made in the last decade, and suggest some of the directions for the future. The Overview provides a brief review of the elements of network survey design—sampling, survey instrument options, network data representation, and network data analysis. There are several good books currently available on the topic of network data analysis, so we provide only a minimal overview here, with suggestions for further readings, and a glossary of network terms used in this volume that may be unfamiliar to the reader. This volume is best used as a guide to the rapidly evolving methodology of network data collection, rather than its analysis. The study chapters are divided up into three groups, reflecting the three basic types of network survey design. These can serve as a guide (and a reality check) for researchers interested in designing network surveys of their own.

Each chapter covers the motivation for the specific project, what worked (and did not work) in terms of survey design and data analysis, and the findings that most clearly represent the insight gained from taking a network approach. The range of design strategies covered here provides a pretty thorough overview of the research methodologies now available for network data collection. The range of findings gives a nice sense of the unique contributions of network analysis to the study of disease diffusion. All of the findings reported here have been published elsewhere in peer-reviewed journals. This was done in order to minimize (again) the need to discuss data analysis methods in detail, preserving the focus on data collection. Interested

readers can consult the cited references to get the full details of the analytic methods
on which the findings are based. We hope the book will serve as a useful reference for
demographers, epidemiologists, network analysts, and formal modelers interested in
the role of networks in disease transmission, migration, and diffusion more generally.

References

Allen, S., Lindan, C., Serufilira, A. et al. (1991). "Human immunodeficiency virus infection in
   urban Rwanda. Demographic and behavioral correlates in a representative sample of childbearing women," *JAMA*, 266(12): 1657–63.

Barabasi, A. L. (2002). *Linked: The New Science of Networks*. Cambridge, MA: Perseus.

Besag, J. (1974). "Spatial interaction and the statistical analysis of lattice systems," *J Royal
   Statist Soc Series B*, 36: 192–236.

Fienberg, S. (1992). "Bibliography on capture–recapture modeling with application to census
   undercount adjustment," *Survey Methodol*, 18: 143–54.

Frank, O. and Snijders, T. A. B. (1994). "Estimating the size of hidden populations using snowball sampling," *Journal of Official Statistics*, 10: 53–67.

—— and Strauss, D. (1986). "Markov graphs," *JASA*, 81: 832–42.

Friedman, S. R., Neaigus, A., Jose, B. et al. (1997). "Sociometric risk networks and HIV risk,"
   Am J Pub Heal, 87(8): 1289–96.

Guimaraes, M., Munoz, A., Boschi-Pinto, C. et al. (1995). "HIV infection among female partners of seropositive men in Brazil. Rio de Janeiro Heterosexual Study Group," *Am J
   Epidemiol*, 142(5): 538–47.

Handcock, M. S. (2003). "Statistical models for social networks: Inference and degeneracy." In
   R. Breiger, K. Carley, and P. Pattison (eds.), *Dynamic Social Network Modeling and Analysis*.
   Washington, DC: National Academy Press.

Heck, R. H. and Thomas, S. L. (2000). *An Introduction to Multilevel Modeling Techniques*.
   Mahwah, NJ: Lawrence Erlbaum Associates.

Hoff, P. D., Raftery, A. E., and Handcock, M. S. (2002). "Latent space approaches to social
   network analysis," *Journal of the American Statistical Association*, 97: 1090–8.

Hook, E. and Regal, R. (1995). "Capture–recapture methods in epidemiology: Methods and
   limitations," *Epidemiologic Rev*, 17(2): 243–64.

Levi-Strauss, C. (1969 [1949]). *The Elementary Structures of Kinship*. Boston: Beacon Press.

Little, R. A. and Rubin, D. B. (2002). *Statistical Analysis with Missing Data*. New York, NY:
   Wiley.

Morris, M. (2003). "Local rules and global properties: Modeling the emergence of network
   structure." In R. Breiger, K. Carley, and P. Pattison (eds.), *Dynamic Social Network Modeling
   and Analysis*. Washington, DC: National Academy Press.

—— and Kretzschmar, M. (1997). "Concurrent partnerships and the spread of HIV," *AIDS*, 11:
   641–8.

Rodrigues, J., Mehendale, S., Shepherd, M. et al. (1995). "Risk factors for HIV infection in people attending clinics for sexually transmitted diseases in India," *BMJ*, 311(7000): 283–6.

Rubin, G., Umbach, D., Shyu, S.-F. et al. (1992). "Using mark-recapture methodology to
   estimate the size of a population at risk for sexually transmitted diseases," *Stat Med*, 11:
   1533–49.

Seber, G. (1982). "A review of estimating animal abundance II," *Int Stat Rev*, 60: 129–66.

Shumway, R. H. and Stoffer, D. S. (2000). *Time Series Analysis and its Applications.* New York: Springer.

Snijders, T. A. B. (2001). "The statistical evaluation of social network dynamics," *Sociological Methodology*, (31): 361–95.

——(2002). "Markov chain Monte Carlo estimation of exponential random graph models," *Journal of Social Structure*, 3(2).

Thompson, S. K. and Frank, O. (2000). "Model-based estimation with link-tracing sampling designs," *Survey Methodol*, 26: 87–98.

——and Seber, G. A. F. (1996). *Adaptive Sampling.* New York: Wiley.

Wasserman, S. and Faust, K. (1994). *Social Network Analysis: Methods and Applications.* Cambridge: Cambridge University Press.

——and Pattison, P. (1996). "Logit models and logistic regressions for social networks: I. An introduction to Markov graphs and p*," *Psychometrika*, 60: 401–26.

Watts, D. (1999). *Small Worlds: The Dynamics of Networks Between Order and Randomness.* Princeton, NJ: Princeton University Press.

——(2003). *Six Degrees: The Science of a Connected Age.* New York: W.W. Norton & Company.

Weniger, B., Limpakarnjanarat, K., Ungchusak, K. et al. (1991). "The epidemiology of HIV infection and AIDS in Thailand." *AIDS*, 5(Suppl 2): S71–85.

Overview of Network Survey Designs

MARTINA MORRIS

A network can be defined as a set of persons and the relationships among them. The joint focus on persons and partnerships is responsible for all of the differences between a network survey and a more traditional survey. It has an impact on sampling, instrument design, and analysis. Each is described below.

NETWORK SAMPLING

Collecting data from a network is similar to collecting data from a population of persons in one sense—there is a range of sampling strategies that stretches from a census, where the population and the sample are identical (sometimes called a saturation sample), to a simple random sample that is meant to be representative of the population. The latter is dramatically less expensive, but requires support from statistical sampling theory to be representative. There is a wide range of sampling theory available for studies in which the individual (be it a person, a household, a firm, etc.) is the unit of analysis. If we want to know what proportion of the population has been immunized against polio, or what proportion of households have at least one child under 6 years old in residence, there are many ways to design an efficient probability sample. This is not to say that the practical implementation of a true probability sample is simple or cheap, but we know what has to be done. When the object of interest is a network structure, however, very little sampling theory is available. Say we wanted to know whether a network was completely connected, or how often a person was likely to be connected (directly or indirectly) to ten or more other persons, or how often partnerships involved persons with more than a 5-year age difference. We know much less about how to design a probability sample for research questions like this. The problem is that we rarely know how to establish the probability that any particular unit (person, partnership, or network component) was selected into the sample (the "inclusion probability"). Without this, there can be no inference from the sample we have to the population of interest.

The key difference between a network study and more traditional behavioral studies is that data are needed on the relationships as well as the persons. This means there are two different sampling units: the individual respondents, and the partnerships. Individuals are still the source of all information, of course, but the information they provide is not limited to their own attributes, it includes data that will help establish the pattern of relationships between them and everyone else. The sampling frames for these two units are therefore nested: first we choose how to sample respondents, and then we choose how to sample partnerships from these respondents. The basic variations in network study designs are derived from the ways in which these two levels are sampled.

The continuum of network sampling design is defined by the type of sample used for selecting respondents.[1] At one end of the continuum is a "saturation sample," or census of the relevant population, and we use the term *complete network design* to describe this approach. Other terms in the literature include sociometric and global network designs. There is no problem of inference here, but the cost is that we must enroll the entire population. At the other end of the continuum is the simple random sample of respondents, and we use the term *local network design* to describe this approach. Another common term in the literature is egocentric design. Here the inclusion probability of respondents is known, but one can anticipate that there will be much less information on the network structures formed by the links in the population. There is clearly a middle ground between these two extremes, and it represents a very wide range of designs that are all based on some kind of link-tracing or "snowball" approach. One starts with a set of initial respondents (or seeds). They nominate partners, and these partners are then also enrolled in the sample. The partners nominate their partners, who are also enrolled, and so on. We use the term *partial network design* to describe this approach.

Of the three designs, the partial network design is the most complex. A wide range of strategies is covered by this heading because after the initial sample is enrolled, there is additional sampling involved at two levels: partners and generations. We can enroll some rather than all of the nominated partners at each generation, and we can trace out some rather than all generations in the population. Enrolling all partners, and all generations gives little control over sample size. The classic snowball sample is a partial network strategy. In this design, all partners of the initial respondent are enrolled, for a set number of generations, typically set a priori. With some information on the typical size of a local network, this design gives some control over final sample size, but we know little about the resulting inclusion probabilities. Another partial network strategy is the standard contact tracing used in public health departments to limit the spread of sexually transmitted infections. In this case, every partner is enrolled in each generation, but only those with infection have their partners enrolled in the subsequent generation. Uninfected individuals are thus endpoints, and the sampling stops when the last set of partners are all uninfected (in theory at least). This strategy is very similar to the "adaptive samples" that are now used in the physical sciences to get efficient estimates of the size of small populations (Thomas and Tucker 1996). It is possible to establish the inclusion probability for each person in a true adaptive sample, but this approach again gives little control over final sample size. Random walks (Klovdahl 1989; Liebow et al. 1995; McGrady et al. 1995), which select a random partner from each generation to enroll are another partial network sampling design.

These three designs—local, partial, and complete—represent the range of strategies available at the level of individual enrollment, and the key differences in network survey design. To a large extent, the portion of the network that is revealed by the sample is determined by which of the respondent sampling strategies is chosen.

---

[1] We take up the sampling of partnerships below.

There is another level of sampling that must be done to identify the links, however, and the way that this is done has different implications for each design.

The fact that we are using a second form of sampling to identify links (or partnerships) is often not appreciated. But a network is defined by the links as much as the nodes. Even if we have a saturation sample of individuals, as we do in the complete network design, our information on the partnerships is limited to what the respondents tell us, and that depends on what we have asked them. This may be the reason that the sampling of links is often not explicitly recognized as part of the network sampling process: it happens in the questionnaire. The nesting of the two sampling units, individuals then partnerships, means that part of the sampling occurs in the context of designing the survey instrument.

SURVEY INSTRUMENT DESIGN

The technique we use to sample the partnerships in the questionnaire is called a "name generator"—the question that is used to elicit and identify partners. It may or may not actually generate the actual names of partners, but it does elicit a set of uniquely identified partners, not just a numeric total. This is what distinguishes a true network instrument from a standard survey instrument. A typical name generator in the context of HIV research might be "Think about the person (or persons) you have had sex with in the past six months, and list their initials here."

There are two parts to every name generator: the relation, and the sampling constraint. The relation in the example above is "sex partner." The sampling constraint is the last 6 months. There are many variations in each, and while there is no comprehensive typology that defines these variations, there are some useful guidelines. The relation can be defined by behavior (like the sexual relation above), role (e.g. siblings, spouses, etc.), or affect (e.g. best friend, someone you fear, etc.). In addition, if using a behavioral generator, the behavior can be actual (someone you did have sex with) or potential (someone you would like to have sex with). The sampling constraint is a stopping rule, it defines how many relations you collect data on. Stopping rules can be numeric (e.g. list up to three sex partners), time-delimited (e.g. sex partners in the last 6 months, first partner, last partner), importance-based (the partner you loved the most) or some combination of these. A partial discussion of these issues can be found in the methodological appendix to Claude Fischer's book, *To Dwell Among Friends* (Fischer 1982).

Name generators are part of the questionnaire, but they are a sampling mechanism in network studies. For the local and complete network designs, they provide the sample of partnerships that will be analyzed. For partial network designs, they also affect the sample of respondents due to the link tracing employed in these designs. Name generators in these studies determine the list of persons eligible to be sampled in each subsequent generation. If we imagine the network survey as a flashlight that shines on certain parts of the network, making them visible, the combination of respondent enrollment and name generator are that flashlight.

In addition to name generators, most network questionnaires will have a set of "name interpreters." These are questions about the nominated partners, and the respondent is asked to answer them for each partner separately. A simple example might be, "How long have you known this person?" Depending on the time available for interviewing, there can be a few name interpreters or many. While the purpose of the name generator is to obtain information on the number and structure of links in the network, the purpose of the name interpreter is to provide information that will help to explain variations in the network structure: In the context of HIV transmission, the interpreters can be used to examine: Are partnerships formed at random or do people target others like themselves? Are sexual partnerships strictly sequential, or do some overlap in time? When someone has two partners at a time, is one of the partnerships likely to be very short term?

Name interpreter questions fall into four general categories:

- partner attributes (e.g. age, race, sex, geographic residence, education, etc.)
- relationship attributes (type of relationship, date of first sex, date of last sex, etc.)
- behavioral repertoire in the relationship (frequency of coitus, use of condoms, etc.)
- the alter adjacency matrix (which of the respondent's partners have a relationship with each other).

Some or all of these categories may be used in any particular study. The thing to remember is that every name interpreter is asked separately for every nominated partner. This means that the number of questions can grow very rapidly. Ten name interpreters become thirty questions if the name generator yields three partners.

The partner attribute questions are important when the partners are not enrolled in the survey. In this case, the information you get from the respondent is all you know about the partner. There is clearly some error introduced by relying on respondent reports of their partners' attributes rather than collecting that information from the partners themselves. But the level of error probably depends on the type of question asked. Above all, it is important to ask questions that the respondent can know the answer to. A respondent can probably tell you whether the partner lives in this neighborhood, or the partner's approximate relative age (e.g. 3 years older or younger), but the respondent may not know whether this partner is having sex with someone else. In the context of HIV-related research, partner attribute information is often used to examine mixing patterns—to see whether there is evidence of assortative or disassortative bias in the patterns of partner selection. For this reason, it is important to ensure that the questions are asked in a way that gives you the same information for both the respondent and the partner.

The relationship characteristics help to identify the intensity and the timing of the partnership. In the context of HIV-related research, questions about timing are perhaps the most critical, as this information is used to establish whether partnerships occur sequentially, or overlap in time. If partnerships are concurrent, the potential for rapid spread through the population is increased. Much more detailed information can also be collected here if there is time. For example, when did the respondent first meet this partner, and where? Do others know about this relationship? The more questions asked, the richer the resulting data for the entire sample of partnerships.

The behavioral repertoire questions may look similar to standard behavioral survey questions, but they differ in one key respect: these questions are now partner-specific. Instead of asking a respondent "how often do you use condoms with your sexual partners," you are asking "how often did/do you use condoms with Fred." Two things are improved by this type of question, the quality of the data, and the level of information it contains. The quality is improved because the question is more specific. Instead of asking the respondent to average their condom use over all partners, you are asking for use with a single partner. The more precise the question, the more accurate the answer. A similar effect is achieved in traditional surveys by asking about condom use at most recent intercourse. The level of information is also increased because you now have data on how condom use varies within person, as well as between person. To say someone "sometimes" uses condoms is a very different statement than to say this person never uses condoms with a spouse, but always uses condoms with commercial partners. Partner-specific behavior permits a more precise identification of the level of risk exposure, and the relational context of behavior. The relational context establishes the social constraints to behavioral change. This is the missing piece of the puzzle in more traditional knowledge, attitudes, and practice surveys: whatever the respondent knows or believes, s/he must negotiate the result with the partner.

The alter adjacency matrix is the most novel of the four name interpreter categories, as it only appears in network studies. Again, it is a link sampling mechanism. The respondent is given a matrix with the IDs of the partners nominated in the rows, and also in the columns. Respondents are then asked to put a check in the cell if the row partner and column partner have the specified relationship (e.g. have shared needles in the last year). This can be a time-consuming exercise, as the respondent must evaluate the question for each pair of partners. With five partners, for example, this requires ten questions, and with ten partners, it rises to forty-five questions.[2] For this reason, the alter adjacency matrix is most often treated as an optional element.

Some network designs typically exclude certain categories of name interpreters, though all include the relationship and behavior categories. With complete networks, for example, it is not necessary to ask about the partner attributes: the partner is also a respondent, so we have their attributes from their self-reports. It is also not necessary to ask about the alter adjacency matrix, as again, we have the partner's own reports of their relations with others. There may be other reasons to include these types of questions in cases where the self-reports make it unnecessary. The most common reason would be to evaluate the accuracy of second hand reporting.

In designing a survey instrument, the key trade-off is between the name generator and the name interpreters. A researcher can collect very little information on a lot of partners, or a great deal of information on a few partners. Typically, there is not enough time to do both. If the purpose of the survey is to provide basic parameters for disease simulation studies, then information should be collected from many partners—little

[2] This assumes the relation asked about is nondirectional, like needle-sharing. If it is directional, like insertive anal intercourse, then the number of questions is twice as many.

information approach is probably preferred. If the purpose is to evaluate options for prevention, then it is probably more important to understand the relational context for the key behaviors, and information should be collected from few partners—in-depth information approach may be preferred.

NETWORK DATA REPRESENTATION

The representation of network data is worth a brief note because the techniques for analyzing it are often based on these forms. Complete network data can be represented in an array called an adjacency matrix: a square matrix with each row and column representing a person in the network, and the cell entry representing a link. Often, this link is simply binary, signifying either presence or absence. For example, if the two persons shared needles in the last 6 months the entry will be 1, and 0 otherwise. But the cell entries can also be valued, and potentially indexed by time. If the relation is undirected, the matrix will be symmetric, but otherwise it may not be. An equivalent representation is an "edgelist." This simply strings the adjacency matrix out into a single vector, indexed by the row and column IDs. When the relation data are binary, the rows with 0's are often deleted from the list.

Partial network data will often be represented in a partitioned array (Frank and Snijders 1994). The first set of rows (and columns) refer to sampled respondents, and the second to nominated but unsampled respondents. This results in four quadrants in the array. The upper left quadrant represents links among the sampled respondents. The two off-diagonal quadrants represent the links between sampled and unsampled respondents. If the relations are undirected, the quadrants will be symmetric. If the relations are directed, the lower left quadrant will be empty. The lower right quadrant represents the relations among unsampled respondents. It is, by definition, empty. Partial network data can also be represented by an edgelist.

Local network data are rarely represented in an adjacency matrix, because so many of the links are missing. Instead, these data are often represented in standard flat file format, with respondents as the unit of analysis, and a set of fields for each partner. Alternatively, they can also be represented in edgelist format. These formats reflect the two sampling levels: individuals and partnerships.

STATISTICAL ANALYSIS OF NETWORK DATA

The techniques available for network analysis vary from simple familiar descriptive statistics, to sophisticated methods for the analysis of dependent data that have their origins in spatial statistics, to a range of specialized non-statistical network measures that are used almost exclusively by social network analysts. The term "network analysis" as it is used in the social network literature typically refers to the latter set of specialized measures. These measures were developed to analyze complete network data, and are largely (though not entirely) focused on summarizing the properties of a fixed network. All of these methods focus on modeling the partnership network, however, not the infectious disease process on the network. This is sometimes a source of confusion, as some mathematical approaches to modeling the disease process on a network treat the system as a directed graph, with transmission flowing across a fixed network from one node to another. In network analysis, the pattern and evolution of the network is itself modeled, without reference to the diffusion of a disease. To understand how a network influences the spread of disease, this network model must be integrated in a second step into a dynamic diffusion model.

What makes network models different from more common methods of statistical analysis in the social sciences is that the observations are dependent in a network. It is not simply that the nodes (or nodal attributes) are dependent—a feature that is clear in the case of infectious disease modeling—but also that the links between nodes may be dependent. In serial monogamy, for example, the dependence is at its most extreme: a link between two nodes ensures the absence of a link between either node and any other node in the population. This feature is known as "dyadic dependence," because the state of one dyad has implications for the state of another. This dependence is not a nuisance parameter, as it is in most spatial statistics applications, it is the main focus of analysis.

As there are multiple levels of analysis in the sampling scheme—individuals, partnerships, and networks—there are multiple methods for analyzing networks. To a large extent, the methods track the sampling scheme employed.

Local network methods

The standard survey sampling strategy that produces local network data eliminates much of the dependence observable in a network. As a result, the statistical methods available for local network data will look familiar to most empirical researchers: tabulations, crosstabs, and various forms of regression. The only difference is that the analyst is now working with multiple levels of analysis: the respondent, the partnership, and possibly larger components (e.g. stars of various sizes).

Respondent level analyses are straightforward. The dependent variable will be a summary function of the local network information, for example, did the respondent have any concurrent partnerships in the last three partners, did s/he have both a commercial and a non-commercial partner in the last 6 months, did s/he use condoms consistently with all partners in the last year, is there spatial heterogeneity in the partners' locations, etc. The independent variables will most often be the respondents' sociodemographic attributes. For example, one might model the likelihood of concurrent partnerships as a function of the age, sex, and marital status of a respondent. One can also use the local network summaries as independent variables, however. For example, one could model the likelihood of spatial heterogeneity in the partner's locations as a function of concurrency. As long as the sampled respondents are independent, standard statistical techniques, linear and logistic regression and their variants, can be used.

Local network data typically contain information on multiple partnerships. These can be disaggregated to form a partnership data set, where each case is a partnership, and respondents with more than one reported partner contribute multiple cases to the data set. The concept is formally analogous to a repeated measure design, where the units become "person-years." In this case, there may be some dependence among the units.

A typical question investigated with the partnership data set is whether the attributes of the respondent are correlated to the attributes of the partner: does like mix with like, for example. If the attributes are discrete (like religion or race), the partnership data can be arrayed as a mixing matrix: attributes of respondents forming the rows, and attributes of the partners forming the columns. If one ignores the dependence induced by multiple partners, the mixing matrix can be analyzed using standard log-linear methods. To capture the dependence, a different technique must be used. It is worth noting that the dependence is an empirical question. If each partnership is effectively the result of the toss of a coin, and the coin is well described by a population model—for example, a general preference for age-matching within a 5-year bracket—then it may not be necessary to include parameters for unobserved individual heterogeneity. If, however, there is additional dependencies induced by repeated observations at the individual level, this can be dealt with by one of the standard models for heterogeneity readily available in the statistical literature—mixed effect models and generalized estimating equations (GEE).

Local network data can also be used to analyze larger components—the size is determined by the number of partners reported by respondents. Each resulting "star" is a component, and can be used in part or in total as a unit of analysis. One disease relevant example is the concurrent partnership triad (the respondent and the two concurrent partners). Cross tabulations remain a useful strategy for this type of analysis. For example, one can cross tabulate relational descriptions of the two partners—the type of relation (spouse, friend, commercial partner, etc.), the length of the relation, the ages of the two partners, etc. These in turn can be broken down by the demographic characteristics of the respondent, or, if there are multiple surveys, by population.

What is typically missing from local network analysis is any network level statistics (e.g. centrality, component size distributions, clique structure, etc.). Given the nature of the data—essentially a set of stars plucked out of the overall network—this constraint is the price paid for the simple sampling strategy. Without making further assumptions, it is difficult to go beyond a mixing matrix and the observed "degree distribution" (the distribution of number of partners) to describe the connectivity structure of the network. If one is willing to make assumptions about the unobserved higher-order properties of the network, however, it is possible to extrapolate from the local network data to a complete network that preserves the observed properties. An example of an analytic extrapolation can be found in Kretzschmar and Morris (1996). They derive a network summary concurrency parameter from the observed degree distribution using a moment generating function.

A general and quite promising approach to extrapolation is to simulate a complete graph from the observed local network data using the recently developed statistical methods for random graphs described below. For example, with an estimate of the degree distribution from data, and assumptions concerning homogeneity (that all persons in the network are drawn from the same degree distribution) and random mixing by degree, the resulting network can be simulated. From this simulated complete network, further analyses can be performed, using the full range of more specialized network analysis methods described below. The simulation model can integrate any information available from the local network data, such as the extent of assortative or disassortative mixing, and the timing and sequence of partnerships. To the extent that the global network properties emerge from local rules such as these, the simulation method can provide a faithful representation of the complete network (Morris 2003).

The range of methods available for analyzing local network data is becoming quite rich, in part because it can borrow more heavily from the standard statistical repertoire than the other network sampling designs, and in part because promising new methods for extrapolation are being developed.

Complete network methods

On the complete network side, there are two, largely independent classes of methods. The first is the set of descriptive methods traditionally regarded as "network analysis" by social network researchers. These methods dominate the field of social network analysis, and comprise a range of techniques for measuring nodal position, summarizing overall structure, and partitioning the network into subgroups. There are a number of textbooks that provide an overview of these methods, and several computer packages for implementing them. The other set of methods is grounded in a statistical framework closely linked to spatial statistics. These methods go by a number of different names—(exponential) random graph models, and P^* are the most common. The approach here is to predict the probability of a link between two persons, as a function of the underlying structure of the network. While these methods began to be developed about the same time as the descriptive methods, they have been much slower to progress. It is only in recent years that fully general models have begun to be developed. As a result there are no textbooks currently available, and reliable general-purpose programs are still some years away.

Descriptive network methods draw inspiration from mathematical graph theory, often using tools from linear algebra to obtain summary measures of clustering and connectivity from the adjacency matrix. These tools provide a rich framework for thinking about networks. A brief look at the measures gives an immediate sense of what differentiates network analysis from sample surveys: the focus is on measures like centrality, "paths" and "walks" that connect nodes, component structure and density, clique-like structure, triad balance, "two-mode" networks linking people to organizations, comparing the overlap in different types of relations, "role algebras" and structural equivalence, and a general mapping of the "social space" revealed by the pattern of relations. Readers familiar with multivariate analysis, especially the techniques of clustering and multidimensional scaling, will recognize some of the methods used in the social space analyses. To the extent that individual nodes are the unit on which measures are calculated, it is their position in the network that is of interest, rather than exogenously measured attributes.

There are a number of textbooks that provide a good introduction to these techniques. One of the most complete is Wasserman and Faust (1993). There are also a number of computer packages now available for implementing this type of analysis. One of the most widely used is UCINET (Borgatti et al. 1999), and a more recent package with more sophisticated tools for network visualization is PAJEK (Batagelj and Pajek 1998).

In the context of these descriptive techniques, statistical inference has been addressed in a limited way. To avoid the independence assumption needed for most likelihood-based methods, analysts have relied instead on resampling techniques such as the bootstrap, jackknife, and permutation tests. Effectively, one simulates the range of possible networks that could arise conditional on certain fixed properties (such as the margins of the adjacency matrix), and calculates the measure of interest for each simulation. This provides a distribution of such estimates, and the observed value can be compared to that distribution.

Statistical models for complete network data, while they have been slow to develop, are now coming into their own. These models represent the network in terms of an exponential random graph, and model the likelihood of the graph as a function of covariates that represent network configurations (links, stars, triangles, etc.). These covariates are intended to capture the dependence among the observed dyads. Holland and Leinhardt (1981) were the first to propose using this modeling approach for networks, noting that it was a natural form because the sufficient statistics were explicitly tied to parameters of interest, like indegree, outdegree, and mutuality. Their "$p1$" model (p is for the probability of the graph) was restricted to these three parameters, which technically corresponds to a model of dyadic independence. More complex models for capturing dyadic dependence—such as a propensity for triangle formation that would induce clustering in the network—were possible in theory, but could not be estimated using the methods available at that time. Some progress began to be made with the development of pseudo-maximum likelihood estimation (PMLE). This led to a series of papers on a simple form of "Markov" network dependence, where two links are dependent if they share a node, (Frank and Strauss 1986), and "$p*$" models for more generalized forms of dependence that create higher order cycles and structured components in a graph (Wasserman and Pattison 1996). The current research in this field seeks to place these models on firmer statistical footing, using Markov Chain Monte Carlo (MCMC) estimation algorithms (Snijders 2002).

These statistical models represent an important advance in network analysis, as they provide a principled framework for estimation and inference. But challenges remain in their implementation. MCMC estimation turns out to be difficult in this context (Handcock 2003). Robust estimation programs are now being developed, but they are in the testing stage. In a few years, however, these methods will become more accessible, and will provide a wide range of new tools to empirical network analysts.

Partial network methods

For partial network data analysis, there is little in the toolbox at this point. If the only aim is to estimate the size of a subpopulation, for example, the number of injection drug-users, there are techniques available. One set relies on the theory of capture–recapture methodology, where an individual can be captured once by the sample, and "recaptured" by being nominated by someone else (Bieleman 1993). Another set of techniques is based on adaptive sampling theory, and relies on link-tracing to the edge units of a cluster (e.g. tracing out until none of the alters have the characteristic of interest) (Thompson and Seber 1996).

The analysis of partial network data is an area in which statistical advances are also being made (Thompson and Frank 2000). But it will be some time before general, accessible analytic tools will be available for empirical researchers.

SUMMARY: STRENGTHS AND WEAKNESSES OF THE DIFFERENT NETWORK SURVEY DESIGNS

Complete network designs remain in many ways the gold standard in this field. Such data require information collected on every person and every relationship in the population at risk. In return, it is not necessary to include partner attributes and the alter adjacency matrix in the survey instrument, which can save some time. In the context of HIV-related research, however, the population at risk is hard to bound.

Partial network data collection also requires persons to identify their partners, so that each partner can be traced and enrolled in the study. Data collection would thus require a question like "tell me the *names* of the people you had sex with in the last X months." Such questions are likely to be viewed as highly intrusive by the respondent. They raise significant issues of privacy and confidentiality for the organizations that collect and store the data (Laumann et al. 1994) (cf. also: Udry, J. R. and Bearman, P. S., *New Methods for New Perspectives on Adolescent Sexual Behavior*. Unpublished manuscript, dated Oct. 3, 1996), and similarly important issues for validity and reliability, as intrusive questions may be met with nondisclosure.

Despite these constraints, there have been several recent studies which have collected some form of complete sexual network data. One is the Adolescent Health Study, a survey of adolescents in high schools across the United States, described in Ch. 8 below. In several of the schools that participated in this study, all of the students in the school were enrolled and asked (among other things) about the persons with whom they had had romantic and sexual relationships in the last 18 months. If these persons attended the same school, they were identified. Except for those partners who did not attend the same school as the respondent, the complete network of sexual relationships among these students was obtained. Less complete forms of network data have been collected for populations of injection drug users (Klovdahl et al. 1994; Neaigus et al. 1994) and a "high risk" group of heterosexuals (Woodhouse et al. 1994, see Ch. 4 below). These studies used snowball sampling schemes which made it possible to uniquely identify a large fraction of within-sample ties, and to use complete network techniques to examine the components, densities, and reachability in these populations.

Recent developments in network sampling and estimation have begun to establish statistical methods for working with a partial network information obtained by link tracing (Klovdahl 1989; Watters and Biernacki 1989; van Meter 1990; Frank and Snijders 1994; Thompson and Seber 1996). The idea is to sample from the complete data so that information on the detailed structural properties is preserved, and statistical inferences can be made. This should provide an important step forward in making complete network modeling more empirically accessible.

Local network data, by contrast, require information collected from a representative sample of respondents. These respondents are asked to describe themselves, their partners, and relationships (Burt 1984; Pattison 1993). No contact tracing is needed, nor are the partners named. The respondent is asked to report a list of attributes for each partner, for example, their age, race, and sex, but the partner, otherwise, remains anonymous. While questions about sexual behavior will always be intrusive, the guarantee of partner anonymity reduces intrusiveness and may increase respondent cooperation. This approach is less expensive and intrusive than contact tracing, and thus more feasible for sensitive questions and large populations (Morris 1995). There are now several completed surveys of sexual behavior that have used local network techniques in countries around the world (Wawer 1990, 1993; Laumann et al. 1994; see Chs. 1, 2, and 3 below).

In general, using a specific number of partners as a stopping rule is preferable to using time limitations, as the time limitations may be invoked during the analysis phase, after the data are collected. Given the severe time constraints in most questionnaires, there is clearly a trade off between the number of partners obtained and the number of questions asked per partner. This trade off should be dictated by the purposes of the survey. Where behavioral understanding is the focus, detail on the partnerships is the key. Where epidemiological projections are the focus, numbers and sequences are more important.

The sampling strategy and reduced intrusiveness of the local network approach gives it a strong advantage for data collection, but the trade off is a loss of information on certain network properties. In addition, there is clearly some error introduced by relying on respondent reports of their partners' attributes rather than collecting that information from the partners themselves. How serious these drawbacks are is an important research question. Compared to the standard respondent-based sexual behavior survey questions, however, local network modules are a substantial improvement. They are sufficient for estimating the mixing matrices and the concurrency patterns described here, and they also provide remarkably rich information on the relational context of sexual behavior.

The application of network concepts and models to the epidemiology of HIV has proven fruitful over the past 15 years. Our ability to model and explore the dynamics of disease transmission through complicated population structures is now substantially improved, and the intervention payoffs are beginning to emerge. While few network-based intervention programs have been fielded at this early stage (Engelgau et al. 1995), network concepts are now widely used in the literature on STI prevention and control (e.g. see, vol. 174 of *The Journal of Infectious Diseases* 1996). The network paradigm has provided an important corrective to individualistic theories of behavioral change by making the partnership the primary unit of analysis. With this simple conceptual shift, it becomes possible to recontextualize sexual relations; to understand sexual behavior as an interaction between partners, instead of an isolated individual act. The methods for network data collection that were developed in sociology over the past two decades have been adapted for surveys of sexual behavior. So there is now a comprehensive body of theory, methods, and data to support network models of epidemiological processes. The result is an analytic framework that provides a concrete, empirical basis for studying negotiation, constraints, power differentials, and the meaning of sexual exchange—as well as variations in the larger network structure which channel the spread of infection.

References

Batagelj, V. and Pajek, A. M. (1998). "Pajek—program for large network analysis," *Connections*, 21(2): 47–57.

Bieleman, B. (ed.) (1993). *Lines Across Europe, Nature and Extent of Cocaine Use in Barcelona, Rotterdam and Turin*. Amsterdam: Swets & Zeitlinger.

Borgatti, S., Everett, M., and Freeman, L. (1999). *UCINET 5.0 Version 1.00 for Windows: Software for Social Network Analysis*. Harvard, MA: Natick Analytic Technologies.

Burt, R. S. (1984). "Network items and the general social survey," *Soc Net*, 6: 293–339.

Engelgau, M. M., Woernle, C., Rolfs, R. et al. (1995). "Control of epidemic early syphilis: The results of an intervention campaign using social networks," *Sex Trans Dis*, 22(4): 203–9.

Fischer, C. S. (1982). *To Dwell Among Friends: Personal Networks in Town and City*. Chicago, IL: University of Chicago Press.

Frank, O. and Snijders, T. (1994). "Estimating the size of hidden populations using snowball sampling," *J Official Stat*, 10: 53–67.

——and Strauss, D. (1986). "Markov graphs," *JASA*, 81: 832–42.

Handcock, M. S. (2003). "Statistical models for social networks: Inference and degeneracy in dynamic social network modeling and analysis." In R. Breiger, K. Carley, and P. Pattison (eds.), *Dynamic Social Network Modeling and Analysis*. Washington, DC: National Academy Press, pp. 229–40.

Holland, P. and Leinhardt, S. (1981). "An exponential family of probability distributions for directed graphs," *JASA*, 77: 33–50.

Klovdahl, A. (1989). "Urban social networks: Some methodological problems and possibilities." In M. Kochen (ed.), *The Small World*. Norwood, NJ: Ablex, pp. 176–210.

Klovdahl, A. S., Potterat, J. J., Woodhouse, D. E. et al. (1994). "Social networks and infectious disease: The Colorado Springs Study," *Soc Sci Med*, 38(1): 79–88.

Kretzschmar, M. and Morris, M. (1996). "Measures of concurrency in networks and the spread of infectious disease," *Math Biosc*, 133: 165–95.

Laumann, E., Gagnon, J., Michael, R. et al. (1994). *The Social Organization of Sexuality*. Chicago, IL: University of Chicago Press.

Liebow, E., McGrady, G., Branch, K., Vera, M., Klovdahl, A., Lovely, R., Mueller, C., and Mann, E. (1995). "Eliciting social network data and ecological model-building: Focus on choice of name generators and administration of random-walk study procedures," *Social Networks*, 17(3–4): 257–72.

McGrady, G. A., Marrow, C., Myers, G., Daniels, M., Vera, M., Mueller, C., Liebow, E., Klovdahl, A., and Lovely, R. (1995). "A note on implementation of a random-walk design to study adolescent social networks," *Social Networks*, 17(3–4): 251–5.

Morris, M. (1995). "Data driven network models for the spread of infectious disease." In D. Mollison (ed.), *Epidemic Models: Their Structure and Relation to Data*, Vol. 5. Cambridge: Cambridge University Press, pp. 302–22.

——(2003). "Local rules and global properties: Modeling the emergence of network structure." In P. Pattison (ed.), *Dynamic Social Network Modeling and Analysis*. Washington, DC: National Academy Press.

Neaigus, A., Friedman, S. R., Curtis, R. et al. (1994). "The relevance of drug injectors social and risk networks for understanding and preventing HIV infection," *Soc Sci Med*, 38(1): 67–78.

Pattison, P. (1993). *Algebraic Models for Social Networks*. Cambridge: Cambridge University Press.

Snijders, Tom A. B. (2002). "A Markov chain Monte Carlo estimation of exponential random graph models," *Journal of Social Structure*, 3(2).

Thomas, J. C. and Tucker, M. J. (1996). "The development and use of the concept of a sexually transmitted disease core," *J Inf Dis*, 174(Suppl 2): S134–43.

Thompson, S. K. and Frank, O. (2000). "Model-based estimation with link-tracing sampling designs," *Survey Methodol*, 26(1): 87–98.

——and Seber, G. A. F. (1996). *Adaptive Sampling*. New York, NY: Wiley.

van Meter, K. (1990). Methodological and design issues: Techniques for assessing the representativeness of snowball samples. In E. Lambert (ed.), *The Collection and Interpretation of Data from Hidden Populations*, NIDA monograph 98. Rockville, MD: National Institute on Drug Abuse.

Wasserman, S. and Faust, K. (1993). *Social Network Analysis: Methods and Applications*. Cambridge, Cambridge University Press.

——and Pattison, P. (1996). "Logit models and logistic regressions for social networks: I. An introduction to Markov graphs and p*," *Psychometrika*, 60: 401–26.

Watters, J. and Biernacki, P. (1989). "Targeted sampling: Options for the study of hidden populations," *Soc Prob*, 36: 416–30.

Wawer, M. J. (1990). Behavioral Research for AIDS Prevention in Thailand. National Institutes of Health Research grant.

——(1993). Ugandan Sexual Network/Behaviors Study for HIV Prevention. National Institutes of Health Research grant.

Woodhouse, D. E., Rothenberg, R. B., Potterat, J. J. et al. (1994). "Mapping a social network of heterosexuals at high risk for HIV infection," *Aids* 8(9): 1331–6.

PART I

LOCAL NETWORK DESIGNS

1

Network Data Collection and its Relevance for the Analysis of STDs: The NHSLS and CHSLS

EDWARD O. LAUMANN, JENNA MAHAY, ANTHONY PAIK, AND YOOSIK YOUM

1.1 INTRODUCTION

The National Health and Social Life Survey (NHSLS) was conducted in the United States in 1992 in order to understand more about how HIV was spread throughout the population at large. The 1980s saw both the introduction of HIV in the United States and a continually rising death toll from AIDS. Yet federal agencies knew little about the specific social patterns through which HIV was transmitted. Unlike other infectious diseases, such as measles or influenza, which spread through casual or indirect contact in any public place, HIV has a critically social component in that it requires the exchange of bodily fluids, most likely to occur through sexual intercourse and needle-sharing. An understanding of sexual networks, then, was necessary for understanding how HIV has spread in the US population, and was critical for understanding how quickly—or slowly—HIV would spread in the future. The research was based on the theory that sexual partnering was far from random, being organized by the social characteristics and the pattern of social contacts of the individuals involved. Thus, the object of the NHSLS was to investigate the social aspects of sexual behavior and the ways in which sexual partner choice and sexual behavior were socially organized.

The findings from the NHSLS were reported in *The Social Organization of Sexuality* (Laumann et al. 1994). The NHSLS allowed the examination of the social organization of sexual behaviors and sexually transmitted disease (STD) transmission on the national level, analyzing differences by social categories such as race and ethnicity, education, age, and religion. Specifically, the NHSLS found that the vast majority of

We gratefully acknowledge the financial support of the Ford Foundation (grant #940-1417) and the National Institute for Child Health and Human Development (#1RO1 HD28356 and #1RO1 HD36963-01) in pursuing this work. We also want to thank the International Union for the Scientific Study of Population (IUSSP) for their financial support in making it possible for us to attend this conference. We especially want to acknowledge our debt to Martina Morris, who was a principal organizer of the conference and provided us with invaluable comments and suggestions in preparing the manuscript for publication. The authors are listed in alphabetical order; all contributed equally in preparing the manuscript.

sexual partnerships originate within tightly circumscribed social settings, resulting in most partnerships comprised of persons with similar characteristics and few partnerships between people with sharply different social characteristics. This study provided a compelling way to think about the entire structure of the population and has been important for understanding sexual network patterns at the national level.

However, while the NHSLS was important for understanding these broad patterns, it must be kept firmly in mind that sexual partnering is fundamentally a local process. Typically, two people must live within reasonable geographic proximity in order to initiate and develop a sexual relationship.[1] People meet each other because they are members of the same social network, neighborhood, organization, or other social entity. Thus, sexual partnering opportunities are heavily structured by the local organization of social life, the local population mix, and the shared norms guiding the types of relationships that are sanctioned or supported. In the NHSLS, it is impossible to investigate the various aspects of social context in any detail because respondents are spread too widely across locales with different norms, opportunities, and supports for various sorts of sexual partnering and practices. In an effort to better understand the local context of social and sexual networks as they actually occurred on the ground, the Chicago Health and Social Life Survey (CHSLS) was conducted in 1995–7.

1.2 SAMPLE

Both the NHSLS and the CHSLS were cross-sectional, population-based surveys. The NHSLS used a national multistage area probability sample designed to give each US household a known probability of inclusion. The interviews were conducted in person with non-institutionalized men and women 18–59 years old. The overall response rate for this survey was 79 percent,[2] yielding a total of 3432 cases, which included over-samples of African Americans and Hispanics in order to allow for more detailed analyses of these subpopulations.

The CHSLS also used a household probability sample of adults age 18–59. However, the CHSLS drew samples at two geographic levels: the city level (including the inner suburban ring) and the neighborhood level (four targeted neighborhood areas within the city of Chicago). The four neighborhood samples were selected in order to provide a set of comparative case studies in which we can study sexual networks. Because this is a study of sexual networks and health, we selected neighborhoods that had

---

[1] However, travelers may behave differently and provide links between separate local networks. And, while it is possible in some cases for two people to meet without being in geographic proximity, such as over the telephone or internet, they must be in geographic proximity in order to have physical contact to transmit an STD.

[2] This response rate is somewhat higher than average for face-to-face, household-based surveys. For example, the General Social Survey successfully interviews about 75% of the target sample, on average Davis, J. A. and Smith, T. W. (1991). *General Social Surveys, 1972–1991: Cumulative Codebook*. Chicago: National Opinion Research Center. Experience shows that such moderately high response rates as 75% do not lead to biased results Laumann, E., Gagnon, J. et al. (1994). *The Social Organization of Sexuality*. Chicago: University of Chicago Press.

a concentration of people in groups of particular relevance. One neighborhood had a concentration of gay men, one was primarily African American, one primarily Mexican-American, and the fourth neighborhood included a mix of Puerto Ricans and Mexican-Americans.[3] The response rate ranged between 60 and 78 percent for the five samples, with a total of 2114 cases.

The response rate was lower than we would have liked in some of the neighborhood samples, but it was not due to non-cooperation from respondents. Rather, cost overruns and a sudden termination of the first field phase resulted in a number of targeted respondents not being interviewed because the interviewing staff had been removed from the field. The CHSLS had initially incurred costly household listing expenditures from purchased listings that were of lower quality than anticipated. To correct the situation, it was necessary to undertake a costly process of making our own listings in several neighborhoods. The low response rate in some of the neighborhoods was due to the abrupt termination of field operations that resulted in many "in-process" interview prospects not being successfully pursued to completed interviews. In fact, no special difficulties were encountered in the field, and interviewers reported no special problems gaining cooperation from respondents. During the second field period, additional cases were collected in three of the four original samples, but not in the predominantly African-American neighborhood of "Southtown." This decision was made because limited funds precluded collecting more cases in all neighborhoods, and the number of completed African-American cases in both the cross-section and Southtown was sufficient to sustain independent analysis. Thus, the judgment was made that limited funds be spent collecting cases from areas where the two other minority populations of interest—Hispanics and gay men—were more prevalent, and we still lacked adequate case counts.

While a number of techniques were used as incentives for participation, none of these were unique to these surveys or to network designs. One technique used to gain compliance was to offer incentive fees, although this was used in a strategic way. For the NHSLS, respondents were not initially offered any money, although a $25 fee was used to convert refusals when needed, and in areas known to be difficult, a fee of $10 was offered at the outset. As time went on and it became clear that sufficient funds were available, all respondents were offered $35 ($10 to complete the household enumeration and $25 to complete the interview). For the CHSLS, a fee of $20 was offered initially, and $50 was used to convert refusals. Other techniques included giving endorsement letters from prominent local and national notables to the interviewers to show respondents. In addition, for the NHSLS, a hotline to the research office at the University of Chicago was set up to allow potential respondents to call in with their concerns.

---

[3] Gay men, African Americans, and Puerto Ricans have disproportionately high rates of AIDS and other sexually transmissible infections (STIs). The Mexican population in Chicago is growing rapidly, which has aggravated tensions surrounding the provision of public services to illegal immigrants at any level and to legal residents in a Spanish-language environment. Further, Chicago is one of the few urban areas where enough Puerto Ricans and Mexicans reside to study both groups separately in the same city. Other studies have repeatedly shown the obfuscation that results when different Hispanic subgroups are lumped together, particularly when the different origin groups being combined live in different parts of the country. Thus, it seemed important to take advantage of Chicago's population mix and select two different Hispanic groups for comparison.

1.3 DATA COLLECTION

Interviews for both of these studies were conducted face-to-face, averaging 90 min per case. The NHSLS was administered verbally using the traditional paper and pencil method, while the CHSLS was administered verbally with the computer-assisted personal interview (CAPI) technology, in which the questionnaire was programmed into laptop computers. Interviewers read the questions that appeared on the screen and entered the respondents' answers directly into the computer. However, both surveys also included self-administered questionnaires (SAQs) for particularly sensitive topics. In the NHSLS a section of the questionnaire was given to the respondent to complete him or herself; the respondent then sealed it in an envelope before returning it to the interviewer. In the CHSLS the laptop computer itself was turned over to the respondent so that he or she could read the questions and enter responses directly into the computer. The computer program was designed so that the interviewer could not see the respondents' answers after the respondent had completed the SAQ.

1.3.1 *Questionnaire design*

The NHSLS and the CHSLS both used an egocentric approach to collect extensive information on sexual networks. The careful enumeration and description of sexual partnerships were at the heart of the NHSLS and the CHSLS, although the two studies collected this information in somewhat different ways. The NHSLS used Life History Calendars to collect information on sexual network partners. Respondents were first asked to list all current and past marital and cohabitational relationships. Respondents were asked: "How many different people have you been married to or lived in a sexual relationship with for a month or more?" They were then asked to list each one by their first name, nickname, initials, or any other way to refer to them, starting with the first marriage or cohabiting partner. Respondents were not asked to give any other identifying information about their partner, such as real name, address, or telephone number. Their partners could remain otherwise anonymous to us, since we would not contact them as in a sociocentric study. The main purpose here was to obtain information about the relevant characteristics of their partners, such as race/ethnicity, age, educational level, and the timing of the relationships.

Next, respondents were asked about sexual partners in the past 12 months. Respondents were given a definition of what constitutes sexual activity (see questionnaire) and were asked "How many people, including men and women, have you had sexual activity with, even if only one time?" The respondent was then asked to give just the first name (or any other way to refer to their partner) of up to nine sexual partners in the last 12 months. Basic information was collected on these sexual partners in the last 12 months, a time period short enough and recent enough to facilitate accurate recall.

The NHSLS then asked more detailed information about the respondent's primary and secondary partner in the last 12 months. The primary partner was defined as either the respondent's spouse/cohabitational partner, or, if they did not have one, the person they considered to be their most important sexual partner in the last year.

If the respondent could not identify one partner that was a primary partner, detailed information was collected on the most recent partner. The secondary partner was defined as the most recent partner in the last 12 months other than the "primary" partner. For these two partners detailed information was collected on the partnering process, sexual practices with the partner, including risky sexual behaviors such as the use of drugs or alcohol during sex, and condom use. Respondents were also asked about their feelings toward their partners and satisfaction with their relationships. And finally, respondents were asked how many partners their partner had in the last 12 months and the concurrency of those relationships with the respondent's relationship. This section included a total of about forty-four questions (varying according to skip patterns), asked of both the primary and secondary partner. Table 1.1 below provides a list of topics covered in the sexual network modules.

The NHSLS then only asked for aggregated demographic information on partners in the last 12 months in excess of these two. Since the vast bulk of the

Table 1.1. *Sexual Network Data in the NHSLS and the CHSLS*

NHSLS

- Number of partners last year, last 5 years, and since age 18
- Timing and demographic characteristics for up to twenty-eight most recent sexual partners
- Marriage, cohabitation, and fertility life histories

- Partnering process information for primary and secondary partners
- Sexual practice data for primary and secondary partners
- Risky sexual behavior (i.e. drugs, alcohol, no condoms) with primary and secondary partners

- Emotional and physical satisfaction with primary and secondary relationships
- Respondents' assessments of primary and secondary partners' sexual activities with other individuals

CHSLS

- Number of partners last year, since age 18, and over the lifetime
- Timing and demographic characteristics for up to five sexual partners last year
- Demographic characteristics of two most recent partners
- Marriage and cohabitation histories with two most recent partners

- Partnering process information for two most recent partners
- Sexual practice data for two most recent partners
- Risky sexual behavior (i.e. drugs, alcohol, no condoms) with two most recent partners
- Emotional and physical satisfaction with two most recent partners

- Household division of labor with two most recent partners
- Relational dynamics with two most recent partners, including embedding among kin and assessments of interpersonal conflict and dependence
- Respondents' assessments of two most recent partners' sexual activities with other individuals

population—80 percent—has only one or no sex partners in a given year, this strategy effectively covers most of the population in an efficient and cost-effective way. From there, the NHSLS turned to a review of the sexual partners since age 18, but phrased it in such a way as to determine partners before, during, and after major relationships (marriages and cohabitations). This technique was an effort to assist recall in reporting partnerships and also served as a way to describe sexual relationships over the life course by organizing the respondent's acquisition of partners around entries and exits from relationships. Using this method, information was collected on up to twenty-eight sexual partners since the age of 18. Finally, respondents were asked basic demographic, relationship, and sexual practice questions about sexual partners before the age of 13, their first sex after the age of 13, and the sexual partners in any forced sexual experiences.

In the CHSLS, extensive sexual network information was simply asked about the two most recent sexual partners, whether or not those partners had been in the last 12 months. The NHSLS data documented that most people's sexual lives are punctuated by periods of more numerous and short-term relationships located between longer and more stable relationships. At any given point in time, most people are in the midst of a longer, more stable relationship; thus, cross-sectional data under-represent more transient partnerships. By collecting information for the two most recent partners, we were able to capture the current primary partnerships of our respondents as well as increase the number of short-term relationships about which we have information. To facilitate administration, the CHSLS instrument was programmed into laptop computers so that logical skips and text substitutions for gender and tense were managed automatically.

The Chicago Health and Social Life Survey respondents were first asked an extensive series of questions about their most recent sexual partner, and then the same set of questions for their second most recent partner. This section totaled approximately seventy-five questions for each partner, but depended on skip patterns. As in the NHSLS, the CHSLS asked basic timing and demographic questions about the respondent's partners, questions about the sexual relationship, sexual practices, and feelings and emotions about the partners and relationship, number of partners their partners had, and concurrency. In addition, however, the CHSLS asked a number of questions about conflict, equity, the household division of labor (if they lived with their partner), and how their lives would be different if they separated from their partner. The CHSLS also asked several spatial network questions. Respondents were asked in which neighborhoods or suburbs respondents' two most recent sexual partners lived. These questions were only asked if the respondent lived in Cook County during the relationship, if the partner was from the last 5 years, and if the respondent did not live with that partner. Respondents were also asked to name a specific place that they go to most often to "hang out," which neighborhood they go to most often to meet potential partners, which neighborhood they work in, and which neighborhoods their friends live in.

If the respondent had more than two sexual partners in the last 12 months, a more limited set of questions was asked for up to three of the remaining sexual partners. These included questions regarding the partners' gender, race/ethnicity, age, and the timing of the relationship. Aggregated information was collected on any remaining partners in the last 12 months. In later sections, respondents were also asked a more limited number of questions about sexual partners before puberty, their first sexual partner after puberty, and then sexual partners since age 18 that had not already been discussed, and finally about anyone who had forced the respondent to have sex.

The main section of the sexual network module took an average of 20–30 min for both surveys, but varied according to the number of sexual partners the respondent had. Answering extensive sexual practice questions for more than a few sexual partners could quickly expand into hundreds of detailed questions, raising issues of recall accuracy as well as making the interview uncomfortably long. So egocentric methods must balance design aspects, which maximize the validity and the reliability of the data, with the informational requirements of the researchers. These questions were at the heart of the alternate designs of the NHSLS and the CHSLS, since each gathered the different types of sex partner information (e.g. timing, demographic, and relationship attributes) with varying levels of comprehensiveness. In general, the NHSLS gathered extensive life-history information regarding the timing and the demographic information of current and past sex partners, while the CHSLS focused more on the relational aspects of the two most recent partners.

In addition to sexual networks, the CHSLS also asked about *social* networks. The social networks in which people are embedded also affect their risk of contracting an STD. Sexual dyads are affected by the social networks surrounding them, and this in turn influences the sexual activity of their members (Laumann et al. 1994). The CHSLS collected information on up to six of the respondents' social network partners. Asking for fewer than six partners can induce an arbitrary list of social network partners because people are forced to choose only a small number of partners (say, three) out of many partners. For egocentric approaches to be effective, elicited network partners must encompass a good part of the entire pool of network partners. The CHSLS first asked respondents to list three partners with whom they spend the most free time, and three partners with whom they discuss important matters. These two lists were merged, removing any duplicate partners. As with the sexual partners, respondents did not have to give the full name of their social network partners, but were instead asked a number of questions about their characteristics, such as race, age, and educational level, as well as their number of sexual partners. Respondents were also asked how each social network partner was related to him or her. This is important since we know that parents have different interests and controls over ego compared to friends, and stepparents may have a very different relationship with ego compared to biological parents.

The CHSLS also asked respondents about the type of relationship between each of their social network partners with each of their other social network partners. The density of the social network ties indicates the extent of the social network's control over ego. In addition, this reveals the diversity of information sources available to ego. The CHSLS also asked respondents whether their social network partners knew either of their two most recent sexual network partners. The relationship between each social network partner and each sexual partner also indicates the extent of control from the social network. In order to ask these complex questions, the

	SX-1	SX-2	SO-1	SO-2	SO-3	SO-4	SO-5
SX-1	N/A						
SX-2	1	N/A					
SO-1	2	1	N/A				
SO-2	1	2	1	N/A			
SO-3	1	1	1	2	N/A		
SO-4	2	2	1	1	3	N/A	
SO-5	2	2	1	2	1	2	N/A

Figure 1.1. *The Matrix-type Questionnaire Prepared by CHSLS*

Note: SX = Sexual Partner; SO = Social Network Partner.

1: Do not know each other; 2: Close friends; 3: Involved in a sexual relationship with one another (not married); 4: Married to one another; 5: Relatives with one another; 6: Friends with one another; 7: Acquaintances.

matrix-form questionnaire in Fig. 1.1 was found useful. It presents one way to ask about the relationship between pairs from the pool of sexual partners and social network partners. We need only half of the matrix because the relationships are symmetric: the relationship between social network partner 1 and social network partner 2 must be the same as one between social network partner 2 and social network partner 1.

1.3.2 Qualitative component

While the national scope of the NHSLS precluded gathering representative qualitative data, the local nature of the CHSLS allowed us to gather valuable qualitative data on the social context of sexual partnering in Chicago. The ethnographic component of the CHSLS consisted of 160 in-depth interviews with community leaders and service providers in four institutional domains where issues of sexual behavior are dealt with. These include: medical, religious, legal, and social services. Staff at agencies located within or serving the populations of our four community areas, or the city of Chicago as a whole, were interviewed about a list of topics including AIDS, other sexually transmitted infections (STIs), domestic violence, homosexuality, family formation, and the like. Interviews lasted between 30 min and 4 h, with most lasting about an hour and a half. Each interview was attended and independently written up by two interviewers for increased completeness and reliability. These interviewers were research assistants hired specifically for this phase of the study, and were not part of the regular National Opinion Research Center (NORC) field staff.[4]

[4] The interviewers for the ethnographic component included four men and four women, two African Americans (one man, one woman), one gay man, one lesbian female, and two persons conversant in Spanish, one fluently. At times these categories were important for gaining cooperation from informants or putting them at ease, and we varied from the prescribed community–institutional specialist pairing when necessary to match interviewers with informants.

1.3.3 Training

Both the NHSLS and CHSLS were conducted by the NORC, and the interviewers for the two surveys were recruited from NORC's field staff and trained as they are for most other surveys conducted by this research center. As with any survey, the interviewers were trained on each section of the questionnaire before entering the field. While the surveys required extensive training for the sensitive nature of the questions regarding sexuality, there was no special training beyond that for administering the network sections.

1.3.4 Confidentiality

The NHSLS and CHSLS raised special concerns about confidentiality both because of the sensitive nature of the questions asked, and because respondents are asked to reveal information not only about themselves, but also about their partners, a special concern when asking questions about HIV/AIDS and other STDs. Two elements of the study design alleviated these concerns. First, because these surveys are cross-sectional rather than longitudinal, all identifying information about the respondent could be destroyed as soon as possible after verification by the NORC central office that the interview had actually taken place. Second, confidentiality of the respondents' partners was less of a concern in the egocentric approach used in these surveys since respondents were not asked to give uniquely identifying information, such as names, addresses, or telephone numbers of their partners. In the sociocentric approach, in which the respondent's network partners must also be contacted by the researcher, such questions are likely to be viewed as highly intrusive by the respondent and therefore met with non-disclosure, raising issues of validity and reliability (Morris 1995).

The fact that the CHSLS was a local study and sampled specific neighborhoods raised another important confidentiality concern, that of making sure the location of the respondents in the four sample neighborhoods cannot be identified. To protect the confidentiality of our respondents in the neighborhood samples, none of the four neighborhoods we sampled correspond exactly to any of the seventy-seven officially designated community areas of Chicago. We have designated each area by a pseudonym, and while it is clear to anyone familiar with Chicago what the general location of each area is, our choice of contiguous tracts with outside boundaries distinct from those of the official areas makes it impossible to know with certainty whether any given census tract falls within one of our sample areas.

1.4 FIELDWORK ISSUES

The network-oriented problems we encountered in the NHSLS and CHSLS were mainly related to the design of some of the network questions, respondents' willingness to list network partners, and questions of mobility in identifying the spatial location of sexual partners.

First, as we have mentioned above, the sexual network modules for the NHSLS and CHSLS were designed to collect detailed information on the timing, number, and relational organization of sexual partnerships. This makes the design and analysis of some of the questions quite complex. For example, in the course of our analyses we found a problem with the design of the questions regarding concurrency, an important determinant in the transmission of STDs. In the CHSLS, the respondent was asked, "To the best of your knowledge, how many people other than you did (partner) have sex with during the course of your relationship?" The fact that no time frame was given for these questions presents a problem for analysis, particularly for relationships of long duration. For example, if the respondent had been in a sexual relationship with the partner for 10 years, we would not be able to distinguish whether the partner's concurrent partnership occurred 9 years ago or just last year. These two possibilities have quite different implications for the respondent's current risk for an STD.

In the NHSLS, on the other hand, a specific time frame was given: "As far as you know, during the past 12 months has (partner) had other sexual partners?" If yes, "About how many partners was that?" The respondent was then asked: "Did (partner) have sex with any of these people during the time you and (partner) were sexually involved?" Of course, in this approach we lose information on the partners' concurrent relationships prior to the last 12 months. The respondent's own concurrency was determined by analyzing the stopping and starting dates for each partnership. This approach presented some problems of its own. To calculate whether or not respondents are currently concurrent in the NHSLS, we had to design an SAS program that checks for overlapping periods for up to twenty-eight partners based on starting and stopping dates of the relationship. There is also additional reliability issues given that respondents were never actually queried whether, say, partner A and partner B actually overlapped, even if the dates indicate concurrency.

A second problem we identified in the course of our analysis was that in the CHSLS, we found that a high percentage of respondents in the Hispanic community in which many illegal immigrants lived did not list any social network partners. Interviewers found that although the respondents were not required to give the actual names or any other identifying information about their network partners, they were reluctant to enumerate their social network partners. The interviewers believed this may have been exacerbated by the fact that we asked those who identified as non-citizens whether they had legal papers. While we thought this question would be valuable in order to understand possible lack of access to regular health-care services and thus lack of diagnosis and treatment of STDs, it remains to be seen whether the cost outweighs the benefit of including this question in the survey. Thus, despite the fact that partners remain anonymous, the egocentric method still requires that researchers be aware of subpopulations that may be particularly reluctant to identify their network partners at all, even with pseudonyms. However, we would expect that if we had asked for their sexual partner's full names and addresses, as required by the sociocentric approach, we would have gained even less cooperation.

Finally, one problem in collecting spatial network data in the CHSLS is that respondents may have moved to their current residence after their relationship with the partner began or ended. Therefore, the respondent's current location does not necessarily reflect their proximity to their partner during their relationship. However, in the CHSLS the geographic questions were only asked of partnerships that took place in the last 5 years. We also asked respondents how long they have lived in the neighborhood, allowing the researcher to assess the degree of mobility and whether this may be a problem in interpreting the results.

1.5 ILLUSTRATIVE FINDINGS

1.5.1 *Second-order connectivity, bridges, and the diffusion of STDs*

The egocentric method used in the NHSLS and CHSLS allows a comparison of the network patterns in different subpopulations of a large population, something that cannot be done with a sociocentric study or an individual-focused survey. Using the NHSLS, Laumann and Youm (1999) found that the differential rates of STIs across racial and ethnic groups can be explained by the different patterns of sexual networks among these groups. The higher prevalence of STDs among African Americans can be explained by examining both the *intraracial* differences between African Americans and other racial/ethnic groups, and the *interracial* patterns of sexual networks between these groups. To determine the intraracial effect, Laumann and Youm (1999) used log-linear analysis to examine how sexual matches between the core, periphery, and adjacent groups within each racial/ethnic group differ across racial/ethnic groups. The relatively high sexual contact between the African-American core group and its periphery facilitates the spread of infection overflow into the entire African-American population. Even though African American in the peripheral group have only one partner (by definition), the chance that their partner is in the core group is five times higher than it is for white peripheral people and four times higher than for Hispanic peripheral people. Therefore, African Americans necessarily have higher infection rates than Whites or Hispanics, even after controlling for number of partners (see Table 1.2).

In addition to this intraracial network effect, Laumann and Youm (1999) also found an interracial effect, which comes from the sexual matching patterns *between* racial/ethnic groups rather than the patterns *within* racial/ethnic groups. From a series of matrix manipulations of the contact matrix simulating different matching patterns between the racial/ethnic groups, Laumann and Youm examined the pure interracial effect, separating its effect from the other confounding effects, such as the differential initial infection rates for each group and the different mean number of partners for each group (Laumann and Youm 1999). From this analysis, Laumann and Youm found that Whites have relatively more sexual contacts with Hispanics than African Americans have. Thus, once infected, Whites can spread infection to other racial/ethnic groups more effectively than African Americans can. Because African Americans are highly segregated from the other racial/ethnic groups in terms of sexual partnering, infections remain within the African-American population. Clearly, these network effects cannot be detected in regressions that include only individual-level risk factors.

Table 1.2. *Contact Matrix (Number of Partnerships for the last 12 months)*

	WP	WA	WC	AP	AA	AC	HP	HA	HC
WP	1463.02								
WA	78.44	199.99							
WC	37.39	160.65	175.98						
AP	12.25	1.53	0.86	172.16					
AA	0.48	3.01	2.16	18.93	67.02				
AC	1.19	5.61	3.91	16.64	59.88	44.93			
HP	33.75	1.91	2.07	2.24	0.39	0.93	82.32		
HA	3.96	4.75	8.25	0.14	1.00	3.66	4.86	9.67	
HC	0.29	4.73	7.79	0.23	2.59	4.32	3.14	13.80	10.41

Note: This table shows the estimated number of partnerships between persons in row (chooser) and column (chosen) groups, calculated according to the procedures described in Appendix A of Laumann and Youm (1999). Since the estimated number of contacts for an ordered row/column combination is the same as for its reversed order, the matrix is symmetric and the upper right-hand entries can thus be omitted to avoid redundancy.
WP: White periphery; WA: White adjacent; WC: White core; AP: African-American periphery; AA: African-American adjacent; AC: African-American core; HP: Hispanic periphery; HA: Hispanic adjacent; HC: Hispanic core.

1.5.2 Concurrent partnerships and the use of condoms

Sexual network data can also be used to investigate how the organization of sexual partnering influences concomitant sex practices. For example, using CHSLS data we can examine the relationship between the structure of concurrent partnerships and how they may impede the use of condoms with sex partners. The CHSLS asked a series of questions on the beginning and ending of sexual partnerships for up to five partners in the last 12 months. These data can be used to identify the structure of egocentric sexual networks in the last year, distinguishing sequential from concurrent partnerships. Among those with overlapping partnerships, we can identify long-term concurrent partnerships as those respondents who had at least two sex partners that overlapped one another for a minimum of 2 months.[5]

Comparing African Americans and Whites, there are discernible differences in the organization of multiple and concurrent partnerships. Only around 8 percent of sexually active Whites, compared to 24 percent of African-American respondents, were involved in at least one concurrent partnership in the last 12 months. Among those with multiple partnerships in the last year, approximately 68 percent of African-American respondents had concurrent partnerships compared to 52 percent among Whites. Moreover, an important difference between African Americans' and Whites' concurrent partnerships is their duration. For Whites, close to 45 percent had

[5] This was necessary since we lacked the specific date of entries and exits to relationships, and we wanted to be sure that the overlapping time period extended at least for 1 month.

overlapping relationships between their first and second partners for less than 2 months.[6] Among African Americans, the period of concurrency is, on average, substantially longer. Only 26 percent of African-American respondents report short-term concurrent relationships. Thus, sexual networks of Whites are mostly monogamous with low levels of long-term concurrency. This patterning of sexual networks reflects a larger partnering process that can be described as sequential monogamy. A substantial proportion of the African-American population, on the other hand, appear to be participating in long-term polygamy, which is primarily organized around nonnuclear couple households and high rates of poverty (Testa et al. 1989).

Furthermore, we can hypothesize that sequential monogamists are likely to adopt condom use as a strategy to reduce risks associated with increased numbers of partners. Individuals in concurrent partnerships, in contrast, particularly long-term ones, are less able to introduce the use of condoms without violating shared norms and trust between sex partners. The results from our ordered logistic regressions strongly confirm this argument. Whites in our analysis are likely to adopt the use of condoms as the risk from multiple partnering increases, but concurrent partnerships do not substantially depress the increasing utilization. In contrast, African Americans involved in long-term concurrent partnerships show a markedly depressed condom use rate even as the risk from multiple partners increases. To facilitate interpretation of our results, we calculated predicted probabilities using the results from the ordered logistic regressions. Figure 1.2 presents the predicted probability of using condoms for an "average person" in our samples. Immediately evident is the impact that concurrency among African Americans has on condom use. The utilization of a condom, in these cases, remains the same regardless of the number of partners and is close to 20 percent lower than for African Americans without concurrent partnerships.

Although we have not directly assessed the importance of long-term concurrency for transmitting STDs, we have provided some evidence about its impact on sexual practices. The infrequent use of condoms, associated with long-term concurrency, is likely to maintain higher infectivity rates among African Americans.

1.5.3 Spatial networks and location of potential bridge areas

The geographic data collected by the CHSLS can be used to better understand the spatial networks through which STDs are transmitted. For example, Mahay and Laumann (2004) have conducted analyses of spatial networks using the CHSLS geographic data. To illustrate the utility of the approach, Fig. 1.3 presents the spatial network data for the four focus community areas in the CHSLS.[7] The solid lines

---

[6] A number of cases have missing data on one of the sex partners. These cases were excluded when calculating the percentage of short-term concurrent partnerships. However, these cases were generally included in the ordered logistic regressions because only information about whether or not the partners overlapped was required.

[7] The four sample community areas are shown on the map as the location of the officially designated community area to which they are closest. However, in order to protect confidentiality, in no case does the community area we sampled exactly correspond to the officially designated area on the map.

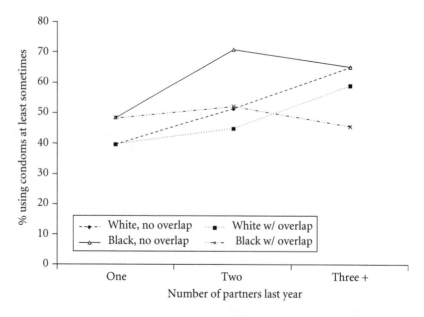

Figure 1.2. *Predicted Probability of Using Condoms By Number of Partners Last Year and Concurrency*

represent the ties between the four focus communities and the community areas in which more than 5 percent of their sexual partners live. The dotted lines represent ties between the four focus communities and the community areas in which between 3 and 5 percent of their sexual partners live. As mentioned above, these percentages are calculated only for single respondents (unmarried and noncohabiting) in each of the four neighborhoods, and are based on the residence of the two most recent sexual partners in the last year. The community areas are shaded according to HIV/AIDS rates.[8]

This map reveals at least two potential bridge communities for the spread of HIV between different areas of the city and different racial/ethnic groups. First, there is a potential bridge area between the gay male population of Shoreland (which has a high HIV/AIDS rate) and the Mexican-American and Puerto Rican populations in Erlinda (which currently has a low HIV/AIDS rate). This area, which lies between these two neighborhoods, is one in which respondents in both Shoreland and Erlinda have sexual partners. A gay club in this bridge area and a park just south of it were mentioned several times by key informants as places where Shoreland residents went to meet partners from other neighborhoods, and where gay men from Erlinda went to find partners because it was safer than remaining in their own community. Thus, the ethnographic evidence suggests that this area acts as a bridge between the White

---

[8] HIV/AIDS data were obtained from the Chicago Department of Public Health, for 1994–6. This time period includes the time when the vast bulk of the CHSLS data were collected.

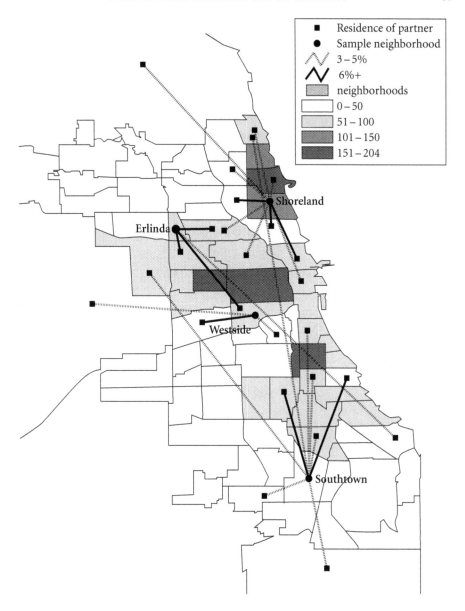

Figure 1.3. *The Spatial Organization of Sexual Partnering*
Source: Laumann et al. (2004).

gay male population and the Latino population, and could lead to the spread of HIV among Latinos.

A second potential bridge area is located on the far north side of the city, where both Shoreland and Southtown (an African-American community with a low

HIV/AIDS rate) respondents have sexual partners. This is a potential bridge area between the White gay male population of Shoreland and the African-American communities on the south side of the city. More analysis must be conducted to examine the degree to which their sexual networks actually overlap. It may be more likely that the spread of HIV to Southtown residents will occur through their sexual contacts with the other African-American communities on the south side that have higher rates of HIV/AIDS (see Fig. 1.3).

These areas are particularly important given the rising rates of HIV infection among heterosexual African Americans and Latinos, increasing the potential for a more widespread transmission of HIV throughout the rest of the population. These bridge communities thus represent places in which resources for the prevention of STD transmission would be most effectively targeted. The analysis of spatial networks is clearly very important for understanding STD transmission. However, it is still a very new area of research, and much more work needs to be done.

1.5.4 Social network effects on the spread of STDs

The CHSLS data on social and sexual networks allow us to analyze the influence that *social* networks have on sexual partnering and STD risk (see Youm and Laumann 2004). Figure 1.4 reveals that there are strong social network effects in addition to those exerted in sexual networks.

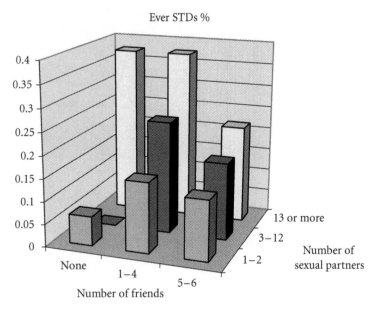

Figure 1.4. *Effects of Social Networks on STDs*

Source: Laumann et al. (2004).

On average, as people have more sexual partners, they are more likely to be infected. However, the effect of having many sexual partners becomes very small among the people who have many social friends. People who have five or six friends have the lowest odds of being infected, once we control for the number of sexual partners (Youm and Laumann 2004). Further analyses will attempt to identify the mechanisms through which these social network effects work, such as whether larger social networks confer an information advantage on their members about the relative risks of potential sex partners or whether larger social networks exert stronger social control over their members with respect to risky partner choice.

These are just several illustrations of the ways in which the types of data collected in the NHSLS and CHSLS can be analyzed to improve understanding of the spread of STDs. These analyses have shown that not only are sexual networks important for the transmission of STDs, but social networks and spatial networks also provide valuable insights into the structure of STD diffusion. Clearly, more work needs to be done on these subjects, and these examples in no way exhaust the types of analyses that can be done with network data. We plan further exploitation of these data, including an analysis of how the relative density of ties between social and sexual networks may affect rates of STD transmission and an analysis of how particular spatial arenas facilitate or hinder the mixing of different demographic subgroups with respect to sexual partner choice.

References

Davis, J. A. and Smith, T. W. (1991). *General Social Surveys, 1972–1991: Cumulative Codebook*. Chicago, IL: National Opinion Research Center.

Laumann, E., Gagnon, J. et al. (1994). *The Social Organization of Sexuality*. Chicago, IL: University of Chicago Press.

——— and Youm, Y. (1999). "Racial/ethnic group differences in the prevalence of sexually transmitted diseases in the United States: A network explanation," *Sex Transm Dis*, 26: 250–61.

Mahay, J. and Laumann, E. O. (2004). "Neighborhoods as sex markets." In E. O. Laumann, J. Ellingson, J. Mahay, A. Paik, and Y. Youm (eds.), *The Sexual Organization of the City* (Chicago: University of Chicago Press).

Morris, M. (1995). "Data driven network models for the spread of infectious disease." In D. Mollison (ed.), *Epidemic Models: Their Structure and Relation to Data*, Vol. 5 (Cambridge: Cambridge University Press), pp. 302–22.

Testa, M., Astone, N. M. et al. (1989). "Employment and marriage among inner-city fathers." *Ann Ameri Acad Pol Social Sci*, 501: 79–91.

Youm, Y. and Laumann, E. O. (2004). "Social networks and sexually transmitted diseases." In E. O. Laumann, J. Ellingson, J. Mahay, A. Paik, and Y. Youm (eds.), *The Sexual Organization of the City* (Chicago: University of Chicago Press).

2

The Thailand and Ugandan Sexual Network Studies

MARTINA MORRIS, MARIA J. WAWER, CHAI PODHISITA, AND
NELSON SEWANKAMBO

2.1 INTRODUCTION

These two network studies were designed and fielded in the early 1990s, with funding from the National Institutes of Health in the United States. The country contexts were (and remain) very different—in terms of economic development, sexual culture and institutions, stage of the epidemic, and public health resources. The local network survey design worked very well in both settings, however, as it had in the United States a year earlier in the National Health and Social Life Survey (NHSLS, see chapter 1).

The questionnaires were structured identically in both studies: information was collected on the three most recent sex partners, with questions on the attributes of the partners, the relationship, and the partner-specific sexual repertoire. This structure was based on the design of a pretest instrument used in the NHSLS. In contrast to the NHSLS (and other) local network studies, however, these two studies did not restrict data collection to partners in the last year—there were no restrictions on the timing of the partnerships. This made it possible to collect data on the sequencing of partnerships, while at the same time preserving the option to restrict analysis to partners in the last year at a later time. The local network items were tailored to the specific context where necessary (e.g. designations for types of partners and for ethnic group), but were otherwise very similar. This standardization of the measurement tool makes it possible to compare the sexual network structures in the two populations—despite some differences in sample design. The partnership networks that became visible through these studies were remarkably different, yet each was efficient for transmission of HIV at the population level in its own way.

Project team—*Principal investigator*: Dr Maria J. Wawer, MD, MPH (Columbia University, USA); *Co-investigators*: Dr Chai Podhisita, Dr Tony Pramualratana (Mahidol University, Thailand); Nelson Sewankambo, MD, David Serwadda, MD (Makere University, Uganda); Martina Morris (University of Washington, USA).

The work reported in this chapter had several sources of funding. Data collection for the two studies was funded by grants from the National Institutes of Health and the Rockefeller Foundation. Data analysis has also been funded by a grant from the National Institute of Child Health and Human Development (R29HD 34957) and the Rockefeller Foundation. The projects involved collaborations between investigators at the Center for Population and Family Health at Columbia University, the Institute for Population and Social Research (IPSR) at Mahidol University in Thailand, and Makerere University in Kampala, Uganda. Programming assistance has been provided by Jeanne Green, Jane Zavisca, Robert Ssengonzi, and Wassana Im-Em over the years.

2.2 THAILAND BRAIDS PROJECT

The Thai project was a single cross-sectional study, carried out from February to December 1992. HIV prevalence in Thailand was rising rapidly at that time in the sentinel surveillance populations of army recruits, sex workers in brothels, and women in antenatal clinics. Thailand had a universal service requirement, so the population of 18–25 year old men in the army was regarded as a nearly complete census of the cohort. Overall prevalence had risen from 2 to 4 percent from 1990 to 1993 among these young men (Shivakumar 2000), and in some of the Northern districts to over 15 percent. The commercial sex industry in Thailand was also quite large at the time of the survey. While some of this industry was driven by a growing international trade in sex tourism, the practice had deep local roots and local patronage. The number of women employed as sex workers was estimated to be about 200,000–300,000 women per year, with potentially as many or more people employed in supportive capacities (Boonchalaksi and Guest 1994). Seroprevalence in the brothels was about 30 percent at the time of the survey. Finally, seroprevalence was rising among pregnant women, from 0.5 percent in 1990 to about 2 percent in 1993, raising fears that a massive epidemic might be in the making, much as it had been in countries like Uganda a few years earlier.

2.2.1 Sample

Quota samples were drawn for three groups: prostitutes working in low-priced brothels, long-haul truck drivers, and low-income men 17–45 years old. Target sample sizes were 500, 300, and 1000, respectively. Completed sample sizes were 678, 330, and 1075. Respondents were sampled in three provinces of Northern and Central Thailand—Saraburi, Udon, and Bangkok—representing semirural, semiurban, and urban settings, respectively. Brothels were chosen from the list compiled by the Ministry of Public Health in each of the three provinces. In each case, the brothel manager was approached to obtain permission to request interviews with the women. If permission was granted, all of the consenting available women in the cooperating brothels were interviewed. Permission was denied in only a handful of cases, and response rates in the cooperating brothels were near 80 percent. Truck drivers were allocated a special over-sample because studies of HIV transmission in other settings had identified this as a high risk group whose mobility had a potentially important impact on the geographic spread of the epidemic. Drivers were interviewed in Saraburi only, at the waiting areas around the two largest cement factories in the country. Thailand was in the middle of a massive building boom, and the cement truck drivers would queue up at these factories for their loads, often waiting for 2 or 3 days as demand outpaced supply. The sample of low-income men was chosen to establish the potential for spread beyond the initial risk groups. These men were sampled in Udon and Bangkok only. Low-income communities were selected from the registry in each region, and a quota sample was drawn from each. Response rates among the truckers and low income men were about 60 percent.

2.2.2 Data collection

Interviewing was done from February to December of 1992. Data were collected using structured interviews, focus groups, and in-depth interviews, and a finger-stick blood sample was taken to test for HIV.

2.2.2.1 Questionnaire

The BRAIDS interview schedule was designed to provide standard sociodemographic data and a range of information on AIDS-related knowledge, attitudes, and sexual behavior. Sexual behavior data were collected in both the traditional summary form, for example, numbers of partners and frequency of behaviors in different time frames, and through a local sexual network module. The network module focused on the respondents' most recent three sexual partners, not restricted by time. Respondents were asked to provide information on the attributes of these partners, the nature and length of the relationship, and the partner-specific sexual behaviors, including the repertoire of sexual activity, condom use, and sex-related alcohol consumption. In all, thirty-two questions were asked about each partner. These are listed in abbreviated form in Appendix 2.1.

2.2.2.2 Qualitative data

The focus group and in-depth interviews were conducted by a smaller set of interviewers, supervised by an experienced local anthropologist. Interviews were transcribed using the program ETHNOGRAPH, and the information was used both independently, and to supplement the quantitative data.

2.2.2.3 Biomarkers

Blood samples were collected on filter paper and tested for HIV for the male sample only. There were many prevalence surveys being conducted among brothel workers at that time, so testing in this study was deemed to be of limited additional value. All samples were initially screened with particle agglutination (Fuji Rebeo, Tokyo) and all positive samples were Western Blot confirmed (Diagnostics Biotechnology, Singapore).

2.2.3 Field experiences

The interviewing staff comprised a small mixed group of experienced and new interviewers. They received minimal training, but were well supervised. The 60 percent survey response rate for the low-income men was lower than one might like, but not unusual for a survey in this context. Among the community men, nonresponse was due primarily to a combination of our inability to contact an eligible household member (after repeated attempts), and to respondents who said they lacked the time to participate. Because these men were likely to refuse before they heard about the topic of the survey, the sensitivity of the topic did not appear to be the driving force in survey nonresponse.

Access to the commercial sex workers (CSWs) required the staff to obtain permission from the brothel managers. In general, this was not a problem. While prostitution was, and is, technically illegal in Thailand, enforcement is rare. The Ministry of Public Health keeps nearly complete records of all brothels and other commercial sex venues, organizing regular testing and treatment for other, curable sexually transmitted diseases (STDs) among sex workers. This system was in place well before the advent of HIV, and it established a precedent for access to the sex workers. This context made it much easier for the survey staff to obtain permission from the brothel manager to conduct interviews, as long as the interviews were conducted outside of working hours. In some cases, of course, the managers did refuse access. Anecdotal evidence suggested that these brothels may have had under-age girls or other problems that they preferred not to reveal.

For the male respondents, the local network questions generated very little non-response from either "don't know" or refusals to answer. The one exception was the education of the partner: respondents did not know the education of about 15 percent of their partners. The great majority (over 85 percent) of the partners for which education was not known were short-term CSWs, so this is probably not a finding that would generalize to other settings. Missing data for other questions about partners typically ranged from 1 to 3 percent, a rate comparable or below that of the non-network survey questions.

For the brothel-based sex workers, virtually all of the last three partners reported were commercial partners. Missing data on these partners was relatively low for some items, like age, region of origin, and economic status, but high (in the 20–40 percent range) for items like education and whether the partner had other partners. Again, given the nature of these partnerships, the high rates of missing data are not surprising, and not generalizable to other settings.

In general, then, the rates of response on the network items were quite high for non-commercial partners. This may be due in part to the effort put in to making the network questions easy for the respondents to answer. We were drawing from a successfully pretested instrument from the US NHSLS (cf. previous chapter in this volume), in which alternative question ordering and wording had been extensively explored. We then worked closely with the local investigators to adapt this instrument to the Thai context. In some cases, however, simplicity for the respondent came at the cost of specificity and detail in the data. A good example of this was in the relationship timing questions. We allowed respondents to answer the question on date of last sex in categories: within last week, last month, last 3 months, last 6 months, 6–11 months, 1, 2, 3, 4, 5, 6–10, and 10+ years. While this may have made it easier for the respondent to answer, it leaves the analyst with much less precision on a key variable. For this reason we changed the questions for the Ugandan survey that followed.

In general, the kinds of problems experienced in the field were those common to all surveys. There was no evidence of problems specifically associated with the network aspects of the survey. In particular, there were very few break offs or refusals to answer the fairly detailed questions in the local network module. The topic of the survey, sexual behavior, did create some problems—not among respondents, however, but among local academics and administrators. As a result, the project investigators were prevented from collecting data from a sample of women in the general population. It was thought that most women would not answer these kinds of questions.

2.2.4 *Illustrative findings from the BRAIDS survey*

Analysis of the BRAIDS data continues, but there are two primary findings that have emerged from the study to date. The first is the overwhelming importance of relational context for determining condom use, even in commercial partnerships (Morris et al. 1995). The second is that "bridge populations" may be as important as "core groups" for the population dynamics of HIV, with important implications for identifying which segments of the population are most at risk (Morris et al. 1996). Both findings could only have been observed using network data and methods.

The Thai government had been promoting 100 percent condom use with commercial sex partners (CSPs) for 2 years prior to our survey. About 50 percent of the men in our survey reported purchasing sex in the last year; among these the median number of commercial partners was five. We found that only 20–30 percent of these men reported consistently using condoms with their CSPs. Among the women who worked in the brothels, about 60 percent reported consistent use. Of the factors found to reduce condom use, the single most important was the relational bond between the partners. If the partner was a "regular" CSP (defined as a partner the respondent has had paid sex with on three or more occasions) the adjusted odds of condom use dropped by 80 percent. The estimate was nearly identical from both the men's and the women's reports.

Among the men, it is the youngest members of the low-income population, 17–24 year olds, that are most likely to report a regular CSP: over 20 percent of those who reported a CSP as one of their last three partners reported a "regular." Because these young men are also likely to report higher numbers of non-commercial partners, their patterns of condom use have important implications for the chain of transmission. Among the women working in brothels, 40 percent report at least one regular in the last three partners, and 20 percent of the last three partners were regulars. Regular CSPs are thus a substantial share of the trade.

Both men and women appear to perceive unprotected sex with regular CSPs as less of a risk for HIV transmission. It seems likely that, as in other sexual partnerships where a personal bond is formed, the sense of emotional safety and trust become an important obstacle to condom use. In focus group and in-depth interviews, the men reported that regular partners know better how to please them, give them better service, and make them feel more comfortable. Perceived safety appears to come both from the sense of control generated by the act of choosing, and from the sense that the "regular" cared for them and would not put them at risk. Among the women working in the brothels, several motives for inconsistent condom use were identified. The first was that condoms imply disease. This is probably very important for women whose livelihood depends on selling sex. The second is that having many regular clients is a source of status among women who work in brothels. The industry encourages stratification, so there is often quite a bit of competition among the workers. It is, of course, nearly impossible for the woman to insist on condom use if the man refuses, unless the brothel manager is willing to back her up. But this is unlikely to be the source of the difference in condom use with casual and regular CSPs. It appears more that regular commercial partners provide a sense of security and comfort for both buyer and seller in the context of paid sex. Under conditions of increasing risk, regular commercial partnerships may become more common, as such partnerships may be perceived as an alternative to consistent condom use or abstinence from commercial sex.

These findings highlight the importance of the relational context of sexual behavior. Individual knowledge and attitudes are necessary to change behavior, but they are not sufficient bases for behavior change once it has to be negotiated with a partner. Relational data, such as that used here, can only be obtained from partner-specific questions in a local network module. As this study shows, it is possible to obtain good basic relational data using appropriately modified survey instruments and standard survey sampling techniques. The quantitative data are made substantially more useful when accompanied by qualitative focus group and in-depth interviews.

The second set of findings from the Thai data were based on an analysis that focused on men who formed a "bridge population" between the women in the commercial sex industry and the women in the general population. We sought to provide a quantitative estimate of the number of women in the general population exposed to the potential for HIV transmission via this bridge. About 17 percent of men and 25 percent of truckers reported both commercial and non-commercial partners in their sexual network during the last 6 months. This was defined as the bridge population for our analysis. Among these men, consistent condom use was less than 30 percent with commercial partners, and effectively zero for non-commercial partners. Extrapolating from the local network data to estimate the rate at which new non-commercial partnerships are formed, we projected that 30 women in the general population were potentially exposed to HIV transmission per 100 sexually active men in the last year, and 9 new women are potentially exposed each additional year. This potential for exposure is only made real if the men become infected with HIV. HIV prevalence in our overall sample of men was low (about 1.2 percent), but men in the bridge population were more likely to be infected with HIV and to have had another STD in the past year (odds ratio 2.2 and 3.5, respectively). Together these figures establish that there was significant potential for HIV to spread into the general population in Thailand. They also demonstrate that bridge populations, such as the men in this sample, can be as important as "core groups" for the spread of HIV.

The patterns of risk and exposure in this analysis suggested three forms of targeted intervention. First, it makes sense to target younger men to promote safer sex. Younger men expose the greatest number of non-commercial partners, so a change in behavior in this group would have greater impact on potential HIV transmission than a similar change among older men. Younger men are also likely to be more receptive to using condoms. They already report higher rates of condom use with both commercial and non-commercial partners—in fact, they were the only group of men to report any consistent condom use with non-commercial partners. Targeting younger men is thus an efficient and effective strategy for intervention.

Second, it is important to target safer sex skills to young women in the general population. The findings here indicated that female peers (non-spousal, non-commercial partners) are exposed in greater numbers than wives. Most of this exposure is created by the youngest men, whose female partners are typically younger than they are. It is critical, therefore, that these young women be informed of the risk they are being exposed to and be given the skills to negotiate safer sex. Both married and unmarried women are clearly at risk here, and the needs of both groups must be addressed. The greater frequency of exposure among unmarried women, however, and the greater likelihood that they, in turn, could infect others, suggests that this population is a more critical link in the system of HIV transmission.

The network data made it possible to demonstrate the importance of bridge populations for the spread of HIV, and to identify more precisely the groups of people who were most at risk. Young men and women are strategic intervention targets because they have more partners, are more likely to be in sexual networks that connect commercial and non-commercial populations, and are more receptive to condom use. It is also likely that in the current context, where the fear of HIV has led to a sharp reduction in commercial sex activity, sexual activity among non-commercial partners may increase, particularly in the younger age groups. Unless condom use increased among non-commercial partners, a change of this sort could actually increase HIV transmission among youth.

As a final note, one of the unanticipated benefits of the local network module was that we were able to obtain a fair amount of information on the partners of our male respondents. Thus, although we were not able to sample women in the general population, we were able to draw a profile of the women whose risk stemmed largely from their partner's behaviors. This is not a complete picture of the women at risk, but it is information we would never have obtained using a non-network survey instrument with the same sample restrictions. While we would not advocate such sample restrictions—they are both inappropriate and ill advised—if one is stuck with them, our experience suggests that a network instrument can mitigate much of the data loss.

2.3 THE UGANDAN SEXUAL NETWORK STUDY

Uganda was one of the first sub-Saharan African countries to experience the full force of the HIV epidemic. Some of the first cases of "Slim Disease" were described in 1985 in the Rakai District where this study was fielded (Serwadda and Mugerwa et al. 1985). By the time this survey was conducted in 1993, HIV prevalence in the major urban sentinel populations in Kampala was nearly 30 percent, and nearly 50 percent of adult mortality in the rural region adjacent to Rakai was estimated to be AIDS-related (Mulder and Nunn et al. 1994). Rakai lies on Uganda's southern border with Tanzania. It is the district through which Tanzanian troops had marched in 1980 to help overthrow Idi Amin, and it also contains a number of key north–south and east–west highways used for transporting goods.

The Ugandan Sexual Networks/Behaviors Study for HIV Prevention (SEXNET) was a 1-year cross-sectional survey inserted into a larger longitudinal study of reproductive health in the Rakai District. The data available from this project has much in common with the Thai BRAIDS study, and also shares key features with the US NHSLS.

2.3.1 Sample

The Uganda SEXNET survey was conducted in ninety communities of Rakai District, using a household-based random sample of 1627 adults aged 15–49. A stratified sampling design was used to guarantee adequate numbers of respondents from rural villages, intermediate villages, and trading centers. Eligible respondents were identified as follows. A village household enumeration was carried out to allocate a unique identification number to each household. On average, villages comprised about seventy households. Using systematic random sampling, twenty-five households were selected per village. A census of the members of selected households was carried out to identify all eligible household members (aged 15–49). A Kish Table (Kish 1995) was then used to select the qualifying member for interview. This gave every eligible member an equal probability of being selected for interview.

The total response rate to interviews in the SEXNET survey was 85 percent, excluding households that did not have any eligible member. There was no replacement of ineligible households. The 15 percent nonresponse includes those who were absent at the time of interview but had qualified for interview during the census, and those who refused to participate in the study. Complete records were not kept on the fraction refusing, but it was estimated by field supervisors to be 8 to 10 percent. The fieldwork period was about 1 year, from November 1993 to December 1994. While focus groups were employed, they were used only to develop the questionnaire.

A number of procedures were adopted to increase validity and reliability. No more than twenty-five persons were interviewed within each community in order to reduce privacy concerns. Interviewers were matched with respondents according to sex, and no other person, especially the spouse, was allowed to be present at the time of interview. While some interviewers were district residents, they were not assigned to interview in their own village, and where such assignments were made inadvertently, the assignment was changed.

While these sample restrictions were adopted as a preventive measure, it should be noted that in a subsequent, much larger study, they were judged to be unnecessary. In the later study all of the households in the community, and all adults in each household were interviewed, though with a much shorter local network module (Wawer et al. 1999).

2.3.2 Data collection

The SEXNET study used a series of focus groups to guide the design of the main questionnaire. No additional qualititative information was collected. Finger-stick blood samples were collected to test for HIV.

2.3.2.1 Questionnaire

The SEXNET instrument collected a wide range of data, including standard socio-demographic information, a lengthy section on travel to and from the mobile markets that circulated around the district, questions on reproductive health, on AIDS-related knowledge, attitudes and beliefs, summary sexual behavior data, and a local network module that focused on the most recent three sexual relationships. As with the Thai survey and the US NHSLS, the local network module contains questions on partner attributes, relationship attributes, and pair-specific behavior between the respondent and each of the three partners. A portion of the local network module was devoted to the last event with each partner. In addition, if respondents had had more than three partners in their lifetime, we collected information on their first sexual partner. In all, seventy-seven questions were asked about each of the most recent three partners (these are outlined in Appendix 2.1). The median interview length was 90 min, though much of this time was devoted to the market module. The detail of the local network questions begins to approach an almost ethnographic quality. For those respondents who had had three or fewer partners in their lifetime (about 50 percent of men and 80 percent of women), we have a remarkably rich picture of their entire sexual history.

2.3.2.2 Biomarkers

All respondents were consented and tested for HIV using blood samples collected on filter paper. Due to technical problems, many of the samples were not properly stored and became unuseable. As a result, these samples have not been analyzed.

2.3.3 Field experiences

As the response rate suggests, the study was remarkably successful. We believe that several factors account for this success. The first was that the study participants recognized the importance of HIV-prevention efforts in their community. Virtually every household had been affected by the epidemic, and the Ugandan government had adopted an active public campaign against AIDS by the early 1990s. As a result, there were lower levels of denial and stigma surrounding the disease, and greater willingness to become involved in prevention-related surveys. The second factor was the long-term presence the project staff had established in this area. The longitudinal survey of reproductive health had been ongoing for 8 years by the time the SEXNET study began. This had a number of beneficial impacts: the staff were well-trained and experienced, the project team had established good working relations with the community, and community residents received benefits from the project over the years. While the project was prohibited on ethical grounds from providing participation incentives to respondents, it had established a local health clinic that benefited all members of the community, regardless of their participation status in any of the project surveys. The final factor was the effort made by the project staff to publicize the purpose of the study and to mobilize community support. Each of the ninety communities selected for the study was visited by the local senior investigators, the study was described, and questions from the residents were answered. In many ways, this study was conducted under ideal circumstances.

In this survey, as in the Thai and US surveys, the item nonresponse for the network questions was quite low. The highest was 8.7 percent, for the partner's village of residence, and the next highest was 7.1 percent for the type of place where the last sex event occurred. For the rest of the questions, about half had nonresponse rates between 1 percent and 2 percent, and half had nonresponse rates below 1 percent. Both men and women in this study provided detailed information on their sexual histories, and their sexual behavior with different partners. There were only a handful of breakoffs. Post hoc it is possible to attribute this to a relatively nonjudgmental sexual culture, in which premarital sexual activity is accepted among both sexes, and polygamy remains common for a minority of men. But this post hoc rationalization bears little resemblance to the concerns that were expressed during the planning stages of the study. In Uganda, as elsewhere, the assumption we had to confront as we embarked on this study was that such "sensitive" data could not be collected in a survey. Our experiences here, as elsewhere, suggest that such concerns are not well founded.

We again aimed to make the items easy for respondents to answer. For example, in this setting, where it is often thought that people have trouble reporting ages, we took care in how we asked the respondent about their partner's age. Rather than asking the respondent to report their partner's age directly, we instead asked the question in two stages. First: "Is [this partner] older or younger than you, or about the same age?" If the answer was older or younger, the respondent was then asked: "About how many years [older/younger]?" Only 2.4 percent of the partner's ages were missing when asked in this way. In addition, even if the respondent could not answer the number of years older/younger, he or she could almost always report whether the partner was older, the same age, or younger—only 0.6 percent of cases were missing this information.

We have some evidence on the validity of the sexual behavior data we collected. There were two places in the questionnaire where the respondents reported the number of sex partners they had ever had: the local network module, and a summary table. The local network module only collected information on four partners (the most recent three, plus the first ever), the summary table recorded the total numbers of partners in the last 6 months, year, and lifetime. We therefore can construct a partial consistency check by comparing these two sources of information, and this is presented in Table 2.1.

For over 98 percent of respondents, the lifetime number of partners reported in the two sections of the questionnaire are consistent. Among the 1.4 percent for whom there is some discrepancy, higher reports on the lifetime summary table is slightly more common. Similar consistency checks can be computed for partners in the last 6 months and the last 12 months. The fraction of respondents reporting consistent numbers of partners in those two time frames in both sections of the questionnaire are 96.2 and 94.8 percent, respectively.

Table 2.1. *Cross Tabulation of the Numbers of Partners Reported in Two Different Sections of the Ugandan Questionnaire*

		Partners reported in summary table					
		0	1	2	3	4+	Total
Partners	0	198	1	0	1	0	200
Reported	1	0	390	1	0	0	391
In Local	2	0	3	357	2	1	363
Network	3	0	0	1	212	7	220
Module	4	0	3	0	2	393	398
Total		198	397	359	217	402	1572

Notes: An additional 3.8 percent answered the summary question saying that they did not know how many partners they had had, and these are not included in this table.

In the analysis phase, we found a few problems with the questionnaire, though they were the types of problems that crop up in any survey. For example, we had neglected to ask whether the respondent expected to have sex with this partner again. This question is important in the analysis of concurrency, because the impact of concurrency depends on the index case alternating sexual partners, and thereby allowing the indirect transmission from each to the other. In practice, we were able to identify whether such alternation had taken place in most cases from other items on the questionnaire. But we would recommend that this question be explicitly included for studies of concurrency.

2.3.4 *Illustrative findings from the Uganda SEXNET study*

As with the Thai survey, analysis of the Ugandan data is ongoing. There have been two primary findings to date. The first concerns the importance of concurrent sexual partnerships for the population dynamics of HIV transmission in Rakai (Morris et al. 1996; Morris and Kretzschmar 2000). The second concerns the importance of travelers in the spread of HIV in this district (Morris et al. 2000).

Concurrent partnerships, that is, partnerships that overlap in time, have been identified as an important behavioral factor that may help to explain the observed HIV prevalence or differentials across populations (Dietz and Tudor 1992; Watts and May 1992; Hudson 1993; Altmann 1995; Morris and Kretzschmar 1995). The intuition for this effect is relatively straightforward. First, from the virus-eye view, there is less time lost after transmission occurs waiting for that partnership to dissolve, or between the end of one partnership and the beginning of another. Second, the effect of partner sequence on exposure risk is reduced. Under serial monogamy each partner increases the risk of infection to a subject, so earlier partners are less likely to be exposed to an infected subject than later ones. If partnerships are concurrent, much of the protective effect of sequence is lost. Earlier partners remain connected to the subject, and are exposed when the subject becomes infected by a later concurrent partner. And finally, concurrency has a critical effect on the "connected component," the number of persons in the population that are directly or indirectly connected at any point in time. Under serial monogamy, the maximum size of a connected component cannot exceed two. Under concurrency, by contrast, the maximum size of a connected component can become quite large: individuals have partners who are themselves connected to others, these others are again connected to additional persons, and so on. Concurrency creates a large, loosely structured, constantly shifting web of connected nodes in a network, enabling an infectious agent to spread rapidly and pervasively. In simulation studies, concurrency has been shown to have very large effects on the spread of a pathogen through a population, raising the growth rate of the epidemic linearly and the prevalence exponentially, even in populations with low rates of partner acquisition. If viremia peaks shortly after infection, the amplification effects of concurrency will be even higher.

This pattern, a relatively low number of lifetime partners but high levels of concurrency, has been shown to be a good description of sexual behavior in the Rakai District of Uganda (Morris et al. 1996; Morris and Kretzschmar 2000). The median number of lifetime partners in this population of 15–49 year olds is 2 for women and 3 for men; the means are 2.5 and 8.4, respectively. This is not a large number of partners. In fact, the distribution of lifetime numbers of partners in this population is similar to that observed in the US NHSLS, and among Thai men in the BRAIDS study (for non-commercial partners). The level of concurrency, however, is quite striking. Nearly 40 percent of the sexually active population reports at least one concurrent partnership among their last three partners; about 55 percent of men and about 27 percent of women. If we restrict the sample to persons with at least two partners in their lifetime—the eligible population—the fraction reporting concurrency rises to 57 percent. Among those reporting at least three partners in their lifetime, 25 percent report that all three of their last three partners were concurrent at some point in time.

The other remarkable aspect of concurrent partnerships in this population is that over 90 percent involve two long-term partners. The most common triad is a respondent with a spouse and a long-term "consensual" partner, slightly over half of all concurrent partnerships take this form. Almost all of the rest are accounted for by polygamy (two spouses), or two long-term consensual partners. This is quite different than the typical "bridge" partnership in the Thai case, where the modal triad will be a man with a long-term partner (often a spouse or girlfriend) and a short-term commercial partner.

There are two important implications of the fact that both partnerships are long term. The first is that the mean overlap for concurrent partners in Rakai is 36 months (95 percent CI, 32–40; IQR, 6–36). This is not determined by the long-term partnerships, but it is only possible with them. The second is that respondents with concurrent partnerships report consistent condom use with at least one of the partners in less than 10 percent of the cases. Consistent use with one partner would be enough to prevent the effective connected component from growing. But condom use with long-term partners is very difficult to sustain. The long overlap between the partnerships involved in concurrency creates the potential for a large, stable, loosely connected network that will amplify the spread of HIV and other sexually transmitted infections.

The difference between partner acquisition rates and levels of concurrency is not simply an academic issue. In populations where the average number of lifetime partners is low but concurrency is common, public health messages that stress the importance of having fewer partners may be ineffective—most people already have few partners, and are unlikely to perceive themselves at risk. For this kind of population, a message stressing the importance of "one partner at a time" is much more important. An effective public health campaign must have accurate information to understand the needs of the specific target population. In this case, a local network module is a simple but necessary tool for collecting the data needed to make an accurate assessment.

The second findings came from an analysis of travelers (Morris et al. 2000), and here we found what appeared to be an effective adaptation to higher risks of exposure to HIV. The population in this district is highly mobile, with over 70 percent reporting travel to a higher prevalence destination in the past year. Travelers are somewhat more likely to have higher levels of sexual partner acquisition, but the risk appears to be offset by significantly greater knowledge, acceptance, and use of condoms. In multivariate analysis, the sexual risk differential for travelers is explained by occupational exposure and higher socioeconomic status. The differential in condom acceptance, by contrast, appears to be associated with travel itself. Condom use with non-spousal partners is three times higher among travelers than non-travelers ($p < 0.001$), and travel remains a significant predictor after controlling age, education, residence, occupation, and multiple partners. Travelers are more likely to use condoms with both their local and non-local partners. This is validated by non-travelers, who report that they are more likely to use condoms when their partners are travelers.

This suggests that something about the experience of travel itself leads to a greater acceptance of condoms. The most likely explanation is that traveling exposes the respondents to new behaviors and weakens traditional social constraints, and thereby helps to lessen the obstacles to condom use. There may also be some influence from exposure to the condom social marketing initiatives, which have targeted the markets and trading centers for several years now. Travelers appear to have learned the importance of safer sex. They represent an opportunity for diffusing behavioral change, not simply spreading the virus. If we ignore this, and see travelers only as disease spreaders, we are missing an opportunity for intervention. For public health systems with limited resources it can be difficult to reach people in rural areas. If prevention programs focus these limited resources on central locations that rural travelers pass through, the travelers can bring their knowledge back to the communities that are more difficult to reach. The Ugandans have a traditional saying for this: "okutambula kulaba, okudda kunyma," roughly, "traveling is seeing, coming back home is telling what you have seen."

With the network module, we were also able to get a detailed picture of the partners of these travelers. This can help to target interventions not simply to respondents who might be at risk, but also to their partners. For example, 49 percent of male travelers report that their non-spousal partners are students and young girls who work at home. This suggests that school-based programs would reach a group of young women who may be at higher risk but whose partners are also more likely to accept a request to use condoms. Among female travelers, 44 percent report that their partners are traders and other blue-collar workers. These partners might best be served by a program targeting markets, hotels, and restaurants. The relatively higher education of women partners in traveler's partnerships may be one of the reasons for the higher rates of condom use. This suggests that women's educational status plays an important role in the dynamics of negotiating safer sex.

We also found that travelers are not more likely to have partners from higher risk occupations when they are on the road, but instead that non-travelers are more likely to have higher risk partners when these partners come from outside the village. This suggests that HIV is introduced into these villages by people from outside, rather than brought back to the village by locals who travel. In part this pattern is probably a function of the study site—a very rural area that in some ways serves as an end-point for the spatial spread of HIV. One would therefore not want to generalize to travelers from all areas. But the patterns do suggest that more careful research is needed to understand the dynamics of HIV spread through spatial networks.

As other studies in this volume also show, the local network module can provide detailed spatial and demographic information on both respondents and their partners. Such data can be used to reconstruct the spatial network of sexual partnerships, and to systematically examine the sexual networks of mobile persons. More systematic study of mobility, and its consequences for both risk enhancement and risk reduction, would make it possible to design intervention programs that disable the network for the spatial spread of HIV.

2.4 SUMMARY

The two studies here provided a remarkably rich increase in information on sexual networks with a relatively small change in survey design: a local network module embedded in a standard survey instrument. With this one small change, we have been able to document many previously unobservable features of the sexual networks in these populations that are important for the spread of HIV. These range from the structural aspects of the sexual network—the "bridge" and concurrent partnerships that are the mechanism for linking partnerships together into components that amplify the spread of HIV (or other sexually transmitted infections)—to the relational context of sexual behavior that puts people at risk of exposure. Both of these studies continue to be analyzed, and much of the current work is comparative in nature. Because the questionnaire designs are so similar, and to the US NHSLS, the comparative analyses are proving to be quite remarkable. On the one hand, the structural features of the network can be compared, and this is beginning to show interesting systematic differences in the networks that either facilitate or impede the rapid spread of HIV. On the other hand, the information on the timing, sequence, context, and content of partnerships is so rich and detailed that one can develop a clear sense of the differences in the culture and organization of sexuality across the different settings.

From the macro to the micro foundations of transmission, the small change in survey design required to collect local network data generates a qualitative increase in the usefulness of the data collected. While the other network survey designs presented in this volume are important for understanding the higher-order properties of sexual networks and their impact on transmission dynamics, the modest local network design has the unique combination of payoff and efficiency needed to become a workhorse in the field of infectious disease epidemiology.

References

Altmann, M. (1995). "Susceptible-infected-removed epidemic models with dynamic partnerships," *J Math Biol*, 33: 661–75.

Boonchalaksi, W. and Guest, P. (1994). Prostitution in Thailand. Phutthamonthon Nakhon Pathom, Thailand: The Institute for Population and Social Research, Mahidol University.

Dietz, K. and Tudor, D. (1992). "Triangles in heterosexual HIV transmission." In N. P. Jewell, K. Kietz, and V. T. Farewell (eds.), *AIDS Epidemiology: Methodological Issues*. Boston, MA: Birkhaeuser, pp. 143–55.

Hudson, C. (1993). "Concurrent partnerships could cause AIDS epidemics," *Int J STD and AIDS*, 4: 349–53.

Kish, L. (1995). *Survey Sampling*. New York, NY: Wiley.

Morris, M. and Kretzschmar, M. (1995). "Concurrent partnerships and transmission dynamics in networks," *Soc Net*, 17: 299–318.

—— and —— (2000). "A micro-simulation study of the effect of concurrent partnerships on HIV spread in Uganda," *Math Pop Stud*, 8(2): 109–33.

——, Pramualratana, A., Podhisita, C., and Wawer, M. (1995). "The relational determinants of condom use with commercial sex partners in Thailand," *AIDS*, 9: 507–15.

——, Podhisita, A., Wawer, M., and Handcock, M. (1996). "Bridge populations in the spread of HIV/AIDS in Thailand," *AIDS*, 11: 1265–71.

——, Serwadda, D. et al. (1996). "Concurrent partnerships and HIV transmission in Uganda." XI International Conference on AIDS, Vancouver, BC.

——, Wawer, M. J. et al. (2000). "Condom acceptance is higher among travelers in Uganda," *Aids*, 14(6): 733–41.

Mulder, D. W., Nunn, A. J. et al. (1994). "Two-year HIV-1-associated mortality in a Ugandan rural population [see comments]," *Lancet*, 343(8904): 1021–3.

Serwadda, D., Mugerwa, R. et al. (1985). "Slim disease: A new disease in Uganda and its association with HTLV-III infection," *Lancet*, 19(Oct): 849–52.

Shivakumar, J. (2000). *Thailand's Response to Aids: Building on Success Confronting the Future*. Bangkok: World Bank.

Watts, C. H. and May, R. M. (1992). "The influence of concurrent partnerships on the dynamics of HIV/AIDS," *Math Biosc*, 108: 89–104.

Wawer, M., Sewankambo, N. et al. (1999). "Control of sexually transmitted diseases for AIDS prevention in Uganda: A randomised community trial. Rakai Project Study Group," *Lancet*, 353(9163): 1522–3.

Appendix 2.1. *Elements on the Thai and Ugandan Local Network Questionnaire Module*

	Partner attributes		Relationship attributes		Sexual behavior		Risk factors
TU	Sex	TU	Type of relationship	TU	Kissing	TU	Condom use
TU	Age	U	Date first met	TU	Fellatio	U	Who brought condom
TU	Race	U	Where first met	TU	Cunnilingus	TU	Other prophylaxis
TU	Ethnic group	TU	Time before first having	TU	Vaginal sex	U	Who chose methods
TU	Village of		sex	TU	Anal sex	U	Astringents in vagina
	residence	TU	Date of first sex	TU	Masturbation	U	Sex during menses
TU	National origin	TU	Date of last sex	U	Forced sex	TU	Respondent alcohol use
TU	Regional origin	N	Expect to have sex again	TU	Other	TU	Partner alcohol use
U	Education	U	Have children with	U	Frequency of sex	TU	Partner's other partners
TU	Occupation	T	Economic support			TU	Number other partners
U	Economic status	U	Cash payments			TU	Type of other partners
U	Alive or dead	U	Relation known to others				
U	Cause of death						

T: Thailand, U: Uganda, N: Neither.

This outlines the question topics for both studies:

- Includes 27 topics for Thailand (indicated by T), 32 actual questionnaire items cited in text.
- 41 topics for Uganda (U), 77 actual quex items cited in text.

3

Sexual Networks and HIV in Four African Populations: The Use of Standardized Behavioral Survey with Biological Markers

MICHAEL CARAËL, JUDITH R. GLYNN, EMMANUEL LAGARDE, AND LINDA MORISON

3.1 INTRODUCTION

Population surveys have a central role to play in the measurement of three of the main determinants of the rate of human immunodeficiency virus (HIV) transmission: age at first sex, number of sexual partners, and use of condoms during sexual intercourse. Measurement of these determinants over time is crucial for the evaluation of prevention programs.

In recognition of that fact, in 1994 the Global Program on AIDS of WHO (GPA) developed a package entitled *Evaluation of a national AIDS programme: a methods package—1. Prevention of HIV infection* Global Programme on AIDS (GPA/WHO). Among the array of methods to measure HIV/AIDS prevention-related indicators, a central place was given to repeated population surveys as a tool for better understanding sexual risk behaviors in the general population and of the impact of

For the Study Group on Heterogeneity of HIV in African cities: Members of the Study Group on Heterogeneity of HIV Epidemics in African cities: A Buvé (coordinator), M Laga, E Van Dyck, W Janssens, L Heyndricks (Institute of Tropical Medicine, Belgium); S Anagonou (Programme National de Lutte contre le SIDA, Benin); M Laourou (Institut National de Statistiques et d'Analyses Economiques, Benin); L Kanhonou (Centre de Recherche en Reproduction Humaine et en Démographie, Benin); Evina Akam, M de Loenzien (Institut de Formation et de Recherche Démographiques, Cameroon); S-C Abega (Université Catholique d'Afrique Centrale, Cameroon); Zekeng (Programme de Lutte contre le SIDA, Cameroon); J Chege (The Population Council, Kenya); V Kimani, J Olenja (University of Nairobi, Kenya); M Kahindo (National AIDS/STD Control Programme, Kenya); F Kaona, R Musonda, T Sukwa (Tropical Diseases Research Centre, Zambia); N Rutenberg (The Population Council, USA); B Auvert, E Lagarde (INSERM U88, France); B Ferry, N Lydié (Centre francais sur la population et le développement, France); R Hayes, L Morison, H Weiss, JR Glynn (London School of Hygiene & Tropical Medicine, UK); NJ Robinson (Glaxo Wellcome, UK); M Caraël (UNAIDS, Switzerland).

The study was supported by the following organizations: UNAIDS, Geneva, Switzerland; European Commission, Directorate General XII, Brussels, Belgium; Agence Nationale de Recherches sur le SIDA/ Ministère français de la coopération, Paris, France; Dfid, London, UK; The Rockefeller Foundation, New York, USA; SIDACTION, Paris, France; Fonds voor Wetenschappelijk Onderzoek, Brussels, Belgium; Glaxo Wellcome, London, UK; BADC, Belgium Development Cooperation, Nairobi, Kenya.

program activities on those risk behaviors. The GPA package gives a comprehensive overview of the design of population surveys and of the necessary steps to be undertaken in the planning of such surveys. There is detailed discussion of objectives; measurement of selected prevention indicators; questionnaire content and design; sampling; training of field staff and collection of data; data management, analysis, and reporting; survey timetables; and in-country survey costs.

The methods package has been used extensively since it was published. More than thirty countries have carried out geographically focused population surveys, while some sixty countries have used other parts of the package, such as the health facility survey for measuring STD management (Mertens et al. 1994; Mehret et al. 1996). Repeated surveys that would allow monitoring of behavior change over time are expected to continue with the support of UNAIDS, co-sponsors, and bilateral and multilateral agencies. National AIDS programs around the world are currently using epidemiological fact sheets in which the prevention indicators are an essential element. Demographic and Health Surveys (DHS) with an AIDS module, and behavioral surveillance surveys (Mills et al. 1998) use the same methodology and may aim for national coverage or be more focused, targeting specific populations at higher risk for HIV.

The questionnaire for the measurement of prevention indicators (WHO/GPA) is divided into eight sections: identification; background characteristics; marriage and regular partnerships; non-regular and commercial sex; condoms; STDs and health issues; knowledge of AIDS; and risk perception, behavior change, and attitudes to persons with HIV/AIDS. The main purpose of the sections on marriage and sexual partners was to measure sexual risk behavior for each individual respondent. The sequence of questions was carefully designed to progress from consideration of marriage to other regular partnerships and finally to more transient and potentially high risk sexual relationships. Clearly, these distinctions are multidimensional and complex. Any comprehensive classification would have to take into account not only the persistence of the relationship over time but also the associated expectations and obligations. A blunt and somewhat oversimplified solution was reached: a regular partner was defined as a person with whom the respondent has a relationship involving sexual intercourse for a period of 12 months or more (including a spouse); anyone else is a non-regular partner. Among non-regular partnerships, a commercial sex encounter was defined as a relationship where sex was exchanged for money and where partners did not know each other (Anderson et al. 1991). The underlying principle was that the concept of non-regular partnerships could be conveyed clearly by interviewers only after careful definition and measurement of regular partnerships.

This questionnaire design has proved to be successful in identifying who was at increased risk of HIV, with what type of behavior and how behaviors change over time. The evaluation surveys have been informative for the development and improvement of HIV/STD prevention strategies (Mehret et al. 1996; Mertens and Caraël 1997).

By 1996–7 it was evident that the spread of HIV has been more rapid and more extensive in some regions/cities than in others. Furthermore, it became obvious that the dynamics of these HIV epidemics were not the same and that differences in time since the introduction of the virus cannot alone explain such discrepancies (Buvé et al. 1995). These large variations are poorly understood. Although numerous studies were conducted on HIV risk factors, the results of these studies were difficult to compare with each other because most studies were not population based and different methodologies were used. The GPA/WHO coordinated surveys, designed for evalua-tion, were limited to simple description of key variables of sexual behavior. However, understanding why, within apparently the same "risk behavior" groups, certain people are more likely to be HIV infected than others requires information on how different individuals are connected via *risk networks*. Indeed, people are put at risk not just by their own behavior but by that of others to whom they are linked in sexual networks. Mathematical models show that different patterns of sexual mixing have widely different implications for the spread of the HIV epidemic (Anderson et al. 1991; Hudson 1993; Morris 1997). If people mix within relatively closed groups—young people with young people, married people only with their spouses or other married people, prostitutes only with a well defined group of individual clients—HIV may spread quickly within some of the groups but will have a limited impact on the pop-ulation as a whole. But if there is much more mixing between groups, young girls with older men, injecting drug users having sex with prostitutes, whose clients have sex with their own wives, for instance, the epidemic may take off slowly but will insinuate itself into many more corners of society. *Bridge populations*, which form a link between otherwise unconnected groups, may be of particular importance for the dynamics of the HIV epidemic by linking low and high risk behavior populations.

This involves a shift to an analytical framework that makes *partnerships* rather than *individuals* the primary unit of analysis (Morris 1997). Individual-based approaches explain behaviors by noting the characteristics of the individual: attitudes, knowledge, socio-demographic variables; while partnership-based approaches try to explain behaviors by noting the characteristics of the relationship: its duration, mutual expec-tations, or gender roles, for example. Ideally, for a better understanding of the nature of these networks, information should be collected on every sexually active person and every relationship in the population at risk. This would require respondents to identify their partners so that each partnership could be uniquely identified. That approach would raise serious issues with regard not only to practicability but also to privacy and confidentiality. By contrast, local network data require only information collected from a representative sample of respondents on selected attributes for each sexual partner in a given period. This is the approach that was proposed in the UNAIDS sexual networks questionnaire in 1997 (UNAIDS 1998).

These principles were used to design a comparative population-based study in four African towns with markedly different levels of HIV infection during 1997 and 1998. The study focused on sexual behavior patterns, other sexually transmit-ted diseases, circumcision status of men, and condom use as factors that could potentially explain the observed differences in HIV prevalence in the four towns. The main aim of the study was to explore whether the differences in HIV levels could be explained by differences in sexual behavior and/or factors influencing the probability of HIV transmission during sexual intercourse.

3.2 SAMPLE

The four sites were selected on the basis of the HIV prevalence among pregnant women and trends over time in this prevalence, aiming for towns where the prevalence had been stable for some years. Other criteria for selection were the local laboratory capacities, local expertise, size of the towns, political stability, etc (Buvé et al. 2001). As high HIV prevalence towns, Kisumu (Kenya) and Ndola (Zambia) were selected. The towns with relatively low HIV prevalence were Cotonou (Benin) and Yaoundé (Cameroon).

Before carrying out these population and sub-population surveys, an anthropological assessment of contextual factors determining the differential spread of HIV was done in each study site. Cultural patterns of sexual behavior, marriage and migration patterns in the general population, and contextual factors such as socio-economic conditions were investigated. These qualitative data were used to develop and pre-test the survey questionnaire. In addition, the same team of anthropologists categorized and carried out the mapping of female sex work settings. The results of the anthropological studies were also used to interpret survey findings.

In each of the towns, households were selected by two-stage cluster sampling: an area stage and a household selection stage. Forty to fifty clusters were selected from the lists of census enumeration areas, which were obtained from the census offices in each country. After listing all the households in each cluster, a random sample of 18–20 households was taken. All men and women aged 15–49 years, who slept in the house the night before the visit by the study team, were eligible for inclusion in the study. A sample size of 1000 men and 1000 women was aimed for. A minimum of two callbacks was made to find the eligible respondent.

3.3 DATA COLLECTION

Households were visited by a team consisting of interviewers and nurses or doctors. After giving their informed verbal consent, study participants were interviewed on their socio-demographic characteristics and sexual behavior, using a standardized questionnaire.

Ethical approval for the study was obtained from the national ethical committee in each of the countries where the study took place, as well as from the ethical committees of the Institute of Tropical Medicine, the London School of Hygiene and Tropical Medicine and the Population Council.

3.3.1 Questionnaire

The questionnaire consists of a short form gathering information about the household of the respondent, then questions for the individual himself or herself: identification, background characteristics (13Q), marriage(s) (21Q), sexual relations with other partners (27Q), and questions relating to sexually transmitted diseases (STDs) and other health issues such as contraception (13Q).

A key issue for local network data collection is the question of how many partnerships to collect information on. The sets of questions designed to collect information on a partner were different depending on whether the partner is spousal or non-spousal. The decision was to ask respondents about their non-regular partnerships in the last 12 months to a maximum of eight relationships, starting with the most recent and going back in time. This figure, based on empirical data in a few countries in the African region, may not be justified everywhere. Information was collected for up to four spousal partners and only when the spousal partnership was current at the time of the interview.

In the local network module, each eligible respondent was asked to report on a list of characteristics about themselves and their partners. No contact tracing was done, nor were the partners named. Box 3.1 shows the characteristics asked about in the questionnaire.

3.3.2 Biomarkers

After the interview study participants were requested to give a blood sample, which was tested for HIV, syphilis, and HSV-2; and a urine sample, which was tested for gonorrhea and chlamydial infection. The detailed procedure has been described elsewhere (Buvé et al. 2001). HIV testing was done anonymously, but linked to the interview data and the results of the other laboratory tests. Study participants who wished to know their HIV serostatus were referred for pre- and post-test counseling and re-testing, free of charge. Study participants with symptoms and/or signs suggestive of STD were immediately treated. Any study participants who were found to have serological evidence of syphilis were traced back and also treated. Men were also interviewed about past and present symptoms of STDs and health-seeking behavior.

Box 3.1. *Attributes Asked About in the Sexual Network Module*
(Adapted from Morris 1997)

Respondent's characteristics	Relationship attributes	Partners' characteristics
Gender	Type of relationship	Gender
Age	Duration of relation	Age
Education	Living arrangement	Education
Literacy	Frequency of sex	Ethnic group
Ethnic group	Use of condoms	Marital status
Religion	Place of first sex	Number of other
Place of origin	Duration of relationship	sexual partners
Place of residence	before first sex	Characteristics of other
Marital status	Ongoing or ended relation	partners
Mobility	Number of sexual acts	
Occupation	Exchange of money	
Age at first marriage		
Age at first sex		
Number of sexual partners		

3.3.3 Qualitative data

In each of the four cities, qualitative data was collected on the types and character-istics of sex workers in different parts of the city (Huygens and Caraël 1998). Following this, all the places where sex work was known to occur were mapped and the number and type of female sex workers (FSWs) present in each place at the time of the visit by the study team were recorded. The maps and the list enabled a sample to be drawn that was representative of the different types of sex workers and the different areas of the city where they worked. Indeed, even a large household survey would not give an adequate representation of sex workers. In Cotonou, Kisumu, and Ndola the places where FSWs worked were randomly selected and all sex workers present at the time of the team visit invited to participate. In Yaoundé sex workers were sampled from different zones with probability proportional to size, and sex workers were contacted via other sex workers. In Cotonou brothel and street-based FSWs were deliberately over-represented in the sample (for the purposes of another study) and this was adjusted for in subsequent analysis. The aim was to obtain a sample size of around 300 sex workers in each city. Following informed consent, interviewer-administered questionnaires were used to collect demographic and socio-economic data, history of sex work, and information on "steady partners" and "clients." Information gathered on clients included: number in the last 24 h, total number in the last week, number city-resident, number of first-time clients, sexual practices, and condom use. FSWs were also invited to attend a specially set up field unit, or a designated health center for a free full genital examination for sexually transmitted infections (STIs). Specimens for STIs were collected and analyzed as for the general population survey.

3.3.4 Field procedures

Fieldwork took place in 1997–8. Interviewer selection and training did not differ greatly from survey procedures of other demographic and social surveys such as DHS. Interviewers were young adults and in all sites female interviewers were used for female respondents. Special attention was paid to in-depth training of interviewers about informed consent, non-judgmental attitudes, confidentiality, and privacy. When presenting themselves and explaining the reason for their visit, interviewers were also trained to explain random selection of households and the meaning of anonymity and confidentiality. The 5-day training emphasized role plays to familiarize interviewers with probing and discussing sexual behavior.

Although it varied slightly from one site to another, the fieldwork was conducted by 4–5 teams of four interviewers—two men and two women—accompanied by a supervisor. On average it took less than 30 min to complete the interview, but the length varied with the specific situation of the respondent. A non-sexually active respondent would be asked only twenty questions. A married person with one spouse and no non-spousal partners would be asked forty six questions. A married respon-dent with two spouses and four non-marital partners would be asked 125 questions, which might take 90 min. The refusal rates on individual questions during the interview process were very low.

3.4 FIELD EXPERIENCES

3.4.1 *Response rates*

The overall response rate for the behavioral data, that is, the response rate at the household level multiplied by the response rate at the individual level, was 96 percent for Cotonou, 81 percent for Yaoundé, 86 percent for Kisumu, and 83 percent for Ndola. The low response rate for Yaoundé, Kisumu, and Ndola, which was seen particularly among the men, was of concern. Most of the nonrespondents were never found at home (refusals were less than 2 percent in all sites). After three calls, the response rate for men was 72 percent for Yaoundé, 72 percent for Kisumu, and 61 percent for Ndola. In Kisumu and Ndola a second round was organized in order to try and retrieve as many men as possible. In Kisumu an additional 85 men were interviewed, in Ndola an additional 110 men, bringing the response rates to 81 and 72 percent, respectively. For these two cities men interviewed after intensified efforts were compared with the men who were interviewed at the first round of the survey, in order to assess biases resulting from nonavailability for interview. In both cities men found after intensified efforts were older and more likely to be married than men interviewed in the main part of the survey.

The differences or lack of differences between men interviewed after intensified efforts and men interviewed in the main part of the survey, can only give some indications about possible biases due to non-response. The data from Ndola suggest that men found later might be more sexually active, but definitive conclusions about the men who were never interviewed and about the non-respondents in Yaoundé cannot be made. Unfortunately, due to logistical constraints, it was not possible to collect blood and urine samples in Kisumu at this second round. In Ndola, there was no significant difference in HIV prevalence among men at the first and second round.

Completed questionnaires for sex workers were obtained for 433 women in Cotonou, 328 in Yaoundé, 300 in Kisumu, and 332 in Ndola. HIV test results were available for 275 (63.5 percent) of these women in Cotonou, 324 (98.8 percent) in Yaoundé, 296 (98.6 percent) in Kisumu, and 324 (97.6 percent) in Ndola.

3.4.2 *Limitations of questions about networks*

Respondents were asked to give the characteristics of each non-spousal partner for up to eight partners in the last 12 months, starting with the most recent. Table 3.1 shows the number of non-spousal partners reported by males and females in each city. Very few men and even fewer women reported more than eight partners.

Obviously where a respondent reported more than eight non-spousal partners the partner characteristics for some of the partners would not have been collected. The combined effect of limiting the detailed data to eight partners, and of a small

Table 3.1. *Percent Distribution of the Reported Number of Non-spousal Partners in the Last 12 Months*

Non-spousal Partners	Cotonou		Yaoundé		Kisumu		Ndola	
	Men	Women	Men	Women	Men	Women	Men	Women
0	56.0	83.0	33.0	55.0	56.0	81.0	68.0	87.0
1–5	43.0	17.0	63.0	44.0	44.0	19.0	31.0	13.0
6–8	0.5	0.0	3.0	0.2	0.4	0.0	0.8	0.0
9+	0.2	0.0	0.7	0.1	0.1	0.0	0.6	0.0
Total cases	1016	1089	967	1111	825	1059	714	1007

percentage of men omitting to give any data for some partners means that if counts of partnership characteristics were made based only on the available data (e.g. counts of contacts in which money is exchanged) then the number of such partnerships would be underestimated by 4 percent for men in Cotonou, 8 percent in Yaoundé, 0.5 percent in Kisumu, and 15 percent in Ndola. Attempts to adjust for the missing partnerships are problematic because assumptions would have to be made about the characteristics of these partnerships. An additional problem is that these estimates are very sensitive to the high number of partners reported by a very small number of men and are therefore imprecisely estimated. For women the loss of information due to the eight-partner limit is negligible.

3.4.3 Missing responses for questions on the characteristics of non-spousal partners in the last 12 months

It was anticipated that some characteristics of some non-spousal partners might not be known so "don't know" categories were included for questions on educational and marital status of the partner, whether the relationship had ended, and whether the partner had other steady, casual, or commercial partners. Where a "don't know" category was included respondents tended to choose this category rather than not giving an answer. Table 3.2 shows the number of "don't know" or "missing" responses for selected questions for each city.

Data on age were more likely to be missing in Ndola and Kisumu than in the other two cities and data on length of the relationship was missing for a large proportion of partnerships in Ndola. The questions on partners of the partner were often unanswered in all cities.

To examine whether respondents experienced "fatigue" or "recall bias" in their answers on partner characteristics, the proportion of "don't know" and missing responses was compared between the first four partners described and the second four. (Test results not shown in Table 3.3.) It is possible that the types of relationships for those with large numbers of partners might have been more casual than those with smaller numbers of partners making the characteristics of the partner less likely

Table 3.2. *Missing Data or "Don't Know" Responses for Questions on the Characteristics of Non-spousal Partners in the Last 12 Months*

Variable	Cotonou		Yaoundé		Kisumu		Ndola	
	Men	Women	Men	Women	Men	Women	Men	Women
Age	1	6	2	2	6	14	21	16
Marital status	2	1	3	2	6	2	4	1
Educational status	14	26	18	19	10	15	23	15
Now ended	5	4	9	7	2	1	<1	1
Relationship length	9	4	<1	2	1	<1	21	32
Condom use last contact	5	0	<1	0	<1	0	<1	0
Money exchanged	<1	0	<1	0	<1	0	0	0
Number of partners of partner	58	52	32	29	21	10	39	37
Partner exchanges money for sex with others	62	62	41	50	45	50	34	38
Total cases	730	216	1575	740	612	250	437	146

to be remembered. Therefore analysis was restricted to those men who reported four or more non-spousal partners (Table 3.3). Women were excluded from the analysis because they reported relatively few non-spousal partners.

Age was reported as missing more frequently for the second four partners in all cities, although this was only statistically significant for Yaoundé. This suggests that missing data on partner characteristics does increase with the number of partners. It is impossible to differentiate between a "fatigue" effect and a "recall bias" effect as the later partnerships should also be the least recent. There were no consistent patterns in missing data for the questions on partners of the partner.

The accuracy and completeness of responses will depend on the skills and training of the interviewers as well as on the knowledge and willingness of the respondents, and this may vary between sites.

3.4.4 Sex worker survey

Methods of identifying and sampling sex workers are likely to influence the characteristics of the sample studied. Qualitative data collected in each city before the survey confirmed that the stigma associated with sex work is so great that women often hide it, and are therefore very difficult to identify for the purposes of a survey. The qualitative data also suggested that "lower class" sex workers were more likely to admit to being sex workers. In Kisumu where sex workers reported less often at least primary education and more often sex work as a major income source as compared with the other sites, it may have affected the true representation of sex worker or reflect the poor socioeconomic conditions of the town (Morison et al. 2001). In the

Table 3.3. *Proportion of "Don't Know" or Missing Responses by Partner Order and Number,*
Among Men who Reported Four or
More Non-spousal Partners in the Last 12 Months

Variable	Cotonou		Yaoundé		Kisumu		Ndola	
	1st 4 partners	2nd 4 partners	1st 4 partners	2nd 4 partners	1st 4 partners	2nd 4 partners	1st 4 partners	2nd 4 partners
Age	0	4	3	11	5	7	22	28
Number of partners of partner	72	75	35	40	27	20	42	50
Partner exchanges money for sex with others	62	67	41	37	43	27	41	41
Total cases	93	24	480	133	77	15	113	32

Note: Partnerships are the unit of analysis.

present survey women were identified at places where sex workers were known to meet clients or were brought to the interviewers by peers. Systematic differences in the women who were missed might have led to biases in some of the summary statistics calculated.

3.5 ILLUSTRATIVE FINDINGS

The overall prevalence of HIV infection in men (including men who denied sexual activity) was 3.4 percent in Cotonou, 4.1 percent in Yaoundé, 19.8 percent in Kisumu, and 23.2 percent in Ndola. For women (including women who denied sexual activity) the respective prevalence rates were 3.5, 7.4, 30.1, and 31.9 percent. In all sites, except Cotonou, the overall HIV prevalence was much higher in women than in men. The most striking contrast was found in the age group 15–19, in Kisumu and Ndola. The prevalence of HIV infection in young men was 3.5 percent in Kisumu and 3.7 percent in Ndola, whereas in young women the prevalence rates were 23.0 and 15.4 percent, respectively. The prevalence of HIV infection among FSW's was 57.5 percent in Cotonou, 33.3 percent in Yaoundé, 74.7 percent in Kisumu, and 68.7 percent in Ndola.

The surveys have produced an extensive data set that has been analyzed to explore the risk factors for HIV within each community, in a standardized way, and the factors that differ between communities that might help to explain their different HIV epidemics. Three examples of analysis will be presented here, all of which use the partnership information but to address very different questions: (*a*) how to measure concurrency and the importance of concurrent partnerships; (*b*) how to identify the clients of prostitutes; and (*c*) how to account for the disparity in HIV prevalence between young men and young women.

3.5.1 Measuring concurrency and examining the role of concurrent partnerships

A growing number of researchers consider that the sexual network structures of a population are critical to the HIV epidemic (Hudson 1996; Garnett and Johnson 1997). In particular, models intended to reproduce partnership formation and HIV transmission dynamics suggest that concurrent partnerships (i.e. having a sexual partnership with more than one person in the same period of time) may enhance HIV spread when compared with consecutive partnerships (Watts and May 1992; Morris and Kretzschmar 1997). However, little is known about the extent to which concurrent partnerships may be of importance in explaining the different patterns of HIV spread in populations, as no comparative population data are available.

We discuss the most relevant measures for characterization of sexual networks with regard to HIV transmission. In addition to being critical to HIV/STD epidemics, these measures should have two main properties: they must be derivable from data from available (or feasible) surveys and they should be relevant to prevention.

The measurement of network structures can be based on either population or individual level indicators, and can be computed either at a given time-point or over a given period of time. Stochastic simulation studies of epidemics within networks have been used to identify those statistical measures most relevant for STD transmission. Ghani et al. (1997) used a logistic regression procedure to test the role of a set of network descriptors on simulated gonorrhoea dissemination (gonorrhoea has often a much shorter duration of infection than HIV and results based on this STD can not be fully extrapolated to HIV) (Ghani et al. 1997). Morris et al. (1996) focused on concurrent partnerships and provided a single measure of concurrency (Kretzschmar and Morris 1996; Morris and Kretzschmar 1997). These studies provide relevant statistical measures and try to link network descriptors and epidemic dynamics: among indicators which apply to populations, the percentage of assortative mixing among high sexual activity groups was suggested by Ghani and co-workers to play a role in gonorrhoea spread. Two other measures of network structure were included in analyses described by Ghani and co-workers. These were the distribution of the "component size" (the size of the largest subset of individuals who are connected together in the same network) and the notion of cohesion that describes the density of connections between individuals.

The authors found that the component size and the cohesion were both associated with the establishment and prevalence of gonorrhoea infection. These two indicators require information on the whole sexual network. Finally, the percentage of mutually non-monogamous pairs (pairs in which both partners have other partners) was also shown by Ghani and co-workers to play a role in the establishment of the epidemic.

Morris and Kretzschmar (1997) proposed a measure of concurrency (*k*) derived from the contact graph representing the whole network of sexual relationships.

This index k measures the fraction of partnerships that are concurrent at a given point in time. It has the property of converging to a simple function of the mean (μ) and variance (σ^2) of the number of partners as the number of individuals grows ($k = \sigma^2/\mu + \mu - 1$). Models showed that concurrency measured by k increases both the intensity and the variability of the intensity of an HIV epidemic and that the final size of the epidemic increases exponentially as k increases. In addition, the authors showed k to be directly and linearly related to the largest connected component size measured at the end of each simulation run.

Among variables applying to individuals, the number of partners at distance 1 (direct partners) and distance 2 (partners of partners) was shown by Ghani et al. to be associated with an individual's risk of gonorrhoea infection. The same authors introduced a measure, called closeness, designed to evaluate the centrality of the location of an individual in a network. One can hypothesize that someone at the edge of a network may not have the same risk of infection as someone more centrally located. The logistic regression analysis showed that the centrality of the position of an individual is of importance for that person's individual risk.

In this study, we have used local network data, that is, data collected at an individual level and both newly developed variables and variables found in the literature to assess the impact of concurrent partnerships. The predictive value of these indicators for HIV epidemics was assessed by comparing their levels among four populations with different HIV prevalences and by comparing their levels between infected and non-infected people (Lagarde et al. 2001).

3.5.1.1 Methods of analysis: Indicators of concurrent partnerships

3.5.1.1.1 Kappa. All participants were asked to provide information on all spousal and non-spousal partnerships of the last 12 months. In particular, dates of formation and dissolution of all partnerships that occurred in the last 12 months were recorded. One exception was spousal partnerships, which were only recorded if ongoing at the time of interview. Spousal partners who had had no sex with the respondent in the last 12 months (according to respondent's declaration) were discounted.

For each respondent, we computed the number of partnerships and their variance at 14 time points in the 12 months preceding the interview. We derived Morris's κ indexes from means and variances and compared them between the sites.

3.5.1.1.2 Duration of overlaps. We computed the duration of all partnership overlaps and summed them for each individual. Mean sums were compared between cities.

3.5.1.1.3 Individual index of concurrency. The information was also used to compute an individual index of concurrency, *iic*, designed to fulfil four criteria: (*a*) *iic* summarizes an individual's propensity to keep or dissolve an on-going partnership before engaging in another one; (*b*) *iic* does not depend on the number of partnerships; (*c*) *iic* does not depend on the length of partnerships; (*d*) the measure covers the 12 months period preceding the interview. For each pair of partnerships declared by a respondent, we computed the actual duration of the overlap d and the expected duration ε given the length of both partnerships (see below for calculation of ε). The ratio d/ε can range from 0 to infinity. We obtained a symmetric measure by computing $r = (d/\varepsilon - 1)/(1 + d/\varepsilon)$. This index r varies between -1 and 1, is null when the duration of the overlap equals that expected by chance, is positive when partnerships are more concurrent than expected, and is negative when partnerships are less concurrent than expected. Finally, the pair-specific indexes, r, are summed for each individual to give an overall individual index of concurrency *iic*. Mean values of *iic* for the different cities were compared.

3.5.1.1.4 Computation details for overlap duration expectancy ε. Let A and B be two partnerships with durations a and b, respectively, centered on time points x and y, respectively. The A and B partnerships are represented by the time intervals $I_x = [x - a/2; x + a/2]$ and $I_y = [y - b/2; y + b/2]$. The observation period is $[0, L]$, where L is 12 months. We assume in what follows that $a \geq b$. Participants were asked to provide information on all partnerships in the last 12 months. We are therefore interested in situations for which I_x and I_y have a non-empty intersection with $[0, L]$. This requires that:

$$(x, y) \in \left[-\frac{a}{2}; L + \frac{a}{2} \right] \times \left[-\frac{b}{2}; L + \frac{b}{2} \right] = \Omega$$

Let $\Omega_i \subset \Omega$ be the subdomain in which $I_x \Omega I_y \neq \phi$ (when A and B overlap):

$$\Omega_i = \left\{ (x;y) \in \Omega; \left| x - y \right| \leq \frac{a}{b} + \frac{b}{2} \right\}$$

The probability that partnerships overlap is

$$p = \frac{|\Omega_i|}{|\Omega|} = \frac{aL + bL + ab}{(L + a)(L + b)}$$

Let us now introduce χ_i the characteristic function of Ω_i ($\chi_i = 1$ inside Ω; 0 outside), and $(x;y)$ the length of $I_c \cap I_y$ whenever it is not empty. The expected duration of overlap is then

$$\varepsilon = \frac{\int_\Omega \chi_i(x;y)\ (x;y)dx\,dy}{|\Omega|}$$

A straightforward calculation gives

$$\varepsilon = \frac{b(aL + ab - b^2/3)}{L^2 + aL = bL + ab}$$

The expected duration of overlap in the case $b \geq a$ is obtained by interchanging a and b.

For partnerships that were still ongoing at the time of interview, the duration of the partnerships was doubled for the computation of ε. Similarly, when an observed overlap covered the time of interview, the observed overlap duration, d, was doubled.

3.5.1.1.5 Proportion of respondents in mutually non-monogamous relationships. We were able to compute the proportion of individuals who where in mutually non-monogamous pairs at the time of interview. This relied on the question addressing the number of partner's partners. Response rates for this ranged from 42 to 79 percent (Table 3.2), which casts some doubt on the accuracy of such an index.

3.5.1.2 Outline of results

Measures of concurrency are given in Table 3.4. The concurrency index k at the time of interview was high in Yaoundé (0.98), intermediate in Kisumu (0.45) and Cotonou (0.33), and low in Ndola (0.26). Among men, the mean sum of duration of overlaps per individual varied from 73 days in Ndola to 271 days in Yaoundé. Among women, the mean sum of duration of overlaps varied from 1 day in Ndola to 52 days in Yaoundé.

The *iic* was computed for each respondent reporting more than one partnership (spousal and/or non-spousal) in the last 12 months. Mean values of *iic* ranged from −0.62 in Ndola to 0.07 in Kisumu. The proportion of individuals engaged in mutually non-monogamous pairs was high in Yaoundé (23.5 percent), low in Ndola and Cotonou (4.5 and 5.8 percent, respectively), and intermediate in Kisumu (12.6 percent).

No correlate could be found between average level of these indicators and level of HIV in the different cities. In addition, there was no evidence that higher measures of *iic* predicted a higher risk of HIV at the individual level.

3.5.1.3. Discussion

3.5.1.3.1 Relevance of computing an individual index. The relevance of computing an individual index that addresses network issues may be questioned. Comparisons made at an individual level should be considered with the assumption that someone with a higher *iic* is more likely, on average, to be in a more connected network. This is not always the case, as, for example, the partners of someone who has several concurrent partners may not have other partners. On average, however, the individual propensity not to dissolve a partnership before engaging in another one is likely to increase the probability of being in a connected sexual network.

3.5.1.3.2 Measure accuracy. Another concern is the accuracy of the estimate of overlap occurrence and length. In addition to the fact that partnership reports are subject to bias due to recollection, social desirability, shyness, interviewer effect and so on, inaccuracies arise since the time the partnership ended is recorded in months (although partnership duration could be measured in days). This led to some uncertainty in calculating overlaps when the starting date of a given partnership was close to the ending date of a previous one. Period measures in months were not able to

Michael Caraël et al.

Table 3.4. *Comparison of Network Descriptors Between Cities*

	Cotonou, Benin	Yaoundé, Cameroon	Kisumu, Kenya	Ndola, Zambia
Number of partners (spouses included) at the time of interview[a]				
Mean	1.14	1.42	1.18	1.06
95% confidence interval	1.11 ; 1.17	1.37 ; 1.46	1.15 ; 1.22	1.03 ; 1.09
N	1022	1425	1208	883
Concurrency index k at interview				
k	0.33	0.98	0.44	0.26
95% confidence interval[b]	0.25 ; 0.43	0.84 ; 1.12	0.35 ; 0.55	0.09 ; 0.47
N	1022	1425	1208	883
Sum of overlaps per person (days)[c]				
Men				
Mean	102	271	117	73
95% confidence interval	82 ; 122	224 ; 318	93 ; 141	24 ; 122
N	738	797	697	538
Women				
Mean	3	52	10	4
95% confidence interval	1 ; 5	39 ; 65	5 ; 14	1 ; 6
N	778	922	848	547
Individual index of concurrency (iic)[d]				
Mean	−0.34	−0.01	0.07	−0.62
95% confidence interval	−0.55 ; −0.13	−0.17 ; 0.15	−0.08 ; 0.22	−1.33 ; −0.09
N	279	649	297	119
% engaged in mutually non-monogamous pairs[a]				
%	5.8	23.5	12.6	4.5
95% confidence interval	4.1 ; 7.5	21.0 ; 26.0	10.1 ; 15.1	2.6 ; 6.3
N	722	1114	680	487
HIV prevalence	3.4	5.9	25.9	28.4

[a] Among those who declared at least one partner at the time of interview.
[b] Computed by the bootstrap method.
[c] Among those ever sexually active.
[d] Among those who declared more than one spousal or non-spousal partner in the last 12 months.

distinguish concurrent partnerships with overlaps of a few days, from serial partnerships with gaps of a few days. To investigate this problem we recomputed *iic* with the constraint that an overlap must last more than a given number of days. This solution is not fully satisfactory as it has the property of eliminating the contribution of short sexual partnerships. A possible solution would be to question respondents on concurrency itself. While measuring the occurrence of concurrency seems feasible using this method, it might be harder to estimate concurrency duration.

3.5.1.3.3 Sexual partnership and sexual behavior. Another important concern is the potential discrepancy between duration of a partnership and duration of a sexual relationship. Although the questionnaire specifically asked for the time interval between the first and last episode of sexual intercourse, respondents take into account many miscellaneous relational events to define their partnership formation and dissolution dates. From the point of view of the virus a partnership starts with the first sexual intercourse and ends with the last one. It may be very difficult to solve this problem, as accurate data on coitus dates are impossible to collect over a long period.

3.5.1.3.4 Relationships with HIV prevalence. All network descriptors that were computed failed to discriminate between populations with high and low levels of HIV infection. In particular, the fraction of partnerships that were concurrent, as measured by the k index proposed by Morris et al. (1996) was not higher in cities with high HIV prevalence. Morris and Kretzschmar (1997) simulated HIV spread among virtual populations with a k index ranging from 0 to 0.67, while k in our surveyed populations ranged from 0.26 to 0.98. This may partly explain why our results are not concordant with simulation results that predict an exponential role of concurrency. It would be interesting to assess simulation outputs when k varies from 0.67 to 0.98. The same simulation also showed that the higher the value of k, the greater the uncertainty in the size of the epidemic at the end of the simulation. This may account for the relatively low HIV prevalence in Yaoundé despite a high value of k. However, k is low in Ndola, which should lead to low uncertainty and low HIV prevalence, but the HIV prevalence was 28.4 percent. Finally, cities ranked differently when k and iic were considered. This could be explained by the fact that iic is an individual index that does not take into account partners of partners while k is intended to describe a feature of the whole network. These two indicators therefore do not reflect the same aspect of concurrency.

3.5.1.3.5 Concurrency and matrimonial system. Both spousal and non-spousal partners were included when computing k and iic. Consequently, matrimonial characteristics may play a part in the explanation of the variations of these indicators. However, we found very similar results when excluding spouses: the four populations ranked in the same order as when spousal partners were included (results not shown). In addition, the population of Cotonou, Benin has the highest level of polygyny, and relatively low values of k and iic.

3.5.1.3.6 Sample size for computation of iic. Among the potential limitations of the study it should be noted that iic was computed for small samples: of the initial sample size of 1819, 2116, 2089, and 1889 respondents in Cotonou, Yaoundé, Kisumu, and Ndola, respectively, only 124, 324, 708, and 313 respondents, respectively, reported more than one spousal or non-spousal partner and answered all questions needed to define the date and duration of partnerships.

3.5.1.3.7 Concurrency and epidemic dynamics. Another concern is that data were collected from populations that have already reached relatively stable levels of HIV infection. Currently reported sexual behavior patterns and concurrency of partnerships may differ from those at the start of the HIV epidemic. People with HIV may have changed their sexual behavior as a result of their disease. In addition, parameters of concurrency may also have been underestimated in cities with high levels of HIV since those who died from AIDS are likely to have had higher than average numbers of partners. Another consequence of the choice of cities is that they are all in a mature phase of their HIV epidemic. Models predict that concurrency impacts on the establishment of HIV epidemics but not on maintaining them, and this may explain why we found no impact of concurrency. However, Yaoundé exhibited the highest level of concurrency and HIV prevalence has been relatively low for many years. According to models, Yaoundé fulfils the criteria for the establishment of a major HIV epidemic, which has not occurred so far.

3.5.2 *Identifying the clients of prostitutes*

The role of commercial sex in facilitating the spread of HIV depends, among other things, on the proportion of the male population who use sex workers and the number and characteristics of the other sexual partners of these clients. The "bridging" role of FSW clients in spreading HIV out to the general population has been studied previously by two methods. The first involves interviewing known clients of FSW (Pickering et al. 1992; Morris et al. 1996; Alary et al. 1999; Vernazza et al. 1999) but this does not give an idea of how prevalent contact with sex workers is within the population. The second method involves trying to identify clients of FSW (mainly using the criteria of whether money was exchanged for sex) from surveys asking males about their sexual partners (Carael et al. 1991). However, the appropriateness of using exchange of money as the criteria for defining contact with sex workers has been in question for some time. The aim of the current analysis was to use the detailed data on non-spousal partners collected during this study to develop better criteria for identifying clients of sex workers, and to examine the number and characteristics of the clients thus defined.

3.5.2.1 *Methods used in the analysis*
Different characteristics of non-spousal partnerships were examined using the survey of approximately 1000 men in each city with the aim of identifying clients of sex workers. Considering the limitations of the different characteristics, a definition of contact with a sex worker based on a combination of these characteristics is proposed. Using this definition the percentage of men having contact with an FSW was calculated and their characteristics were described.

The derived definition of contact with sex workers was then used to calculate the total number of FSW partners per 1000 males per year. This was multiplied by the average number of times each man reported intercourse with each FSW partner to estimate total sexual contacts per 1000 men per year. An upper and lower limit was calculated to account for non-spousal relationships for which the characteristics were not available. The lower limit assumes none were contacts with sex workers while the upper limit assumes that all were.

The data from the survey of sex workers were then used to calculate the average number of contacts between sex workers and clients per 1000 men per year. First the annual number of contacts with city-resident clients for each FSW was estimated by multiplying the mean weekly number of city-resident clients by the average number of weeks a FSW was resident in the city. The number of FSW contacts per 1000 men per year was estimated by multiplying the annual number of contacts by the number of FSWs per 1000 men.

3.5.2.2 *Outline of results*

The following characteristics of non-spousal partners of men were examined for use in identifying clients of sex workers: local term used to describe the relationship; exchange of money (always or often) for sex; how long he had known the partner before having sex; the duration of the relationship; the number of partners of the partner; and whether the partner was thought to have sex with others in exchange for money.

Men rarely described non-spousal partners as prostitutes (between 0.4 and 1.8 percent reported sex with a prostitute) limiting the use of this in identifying clients. Table 3.5 shows the proportion of relationships where money was always or often exchanged by type of relationship as described in local terms. The exchange of money occurred between couples engaged to be married, and was not always exchanged in relationships described as sex work.

Therefore exchange of money was combined with other characteristics of the relationship in defining contact with a sex worker. The number of partners of the female partner, and whether the female partner exchanged sex with others for money were considered to be useful criteria for defining contact with a sex worker. However, Table 3.3 shows that a large proportion of responses for these questions had missing answers or the man reported that he did not know. Other possible useful characteristics included whether the relationship had duration of a day or less and whether the partners had sex on the same day they met. There was little missing data for these two characteristics. After considering the limitations of the different questions, the definition of contact with a FSW shown in Box 3.2 was derived.

Table 3.5 shows the local term used to describe relationships, which were defined as sex work according to Box 3.2. Most were described as casual relationships or

Box 3.2. *Definition of Contact with an FSW*

Male partner defined it as a sex work contact *or* it was a relationship where money was always or often exchanged and $\geq$ one of the following:

- duration of 1 day or less
- they had sex on the same day they met
- the female partner was reported to have more than nine partners
- the female partner was reported to exchange sex for money with others.

Table 3.5. *Proportion of "Sex Work Contacts" of Men in the Last 12 Months, Compared with Local Terms Used by Respondents to describe relationship*

	% (*n*)			
	Cotonou	Yaoundé	Kisumu	Ndola
Money always or often exchanged among:				
Fiancée	0 (52)	[a]	17 (12)	44 (16)
Girlfriend	7 (527)	11 (1124)	15 (378)	45 (312)
Casual	36 (119)	43 (387)	20 (198)	42 (105)
Prostitute	71 (24)	72 (36)	50 (4)	25 (4)
Definition of contact with an FSW (Box 2)				
Fiancée	0 (52)	[a]	0 (12)	0 (16)
Girlfriend	1 (530)	6 (1127)	4 (361)	14 (312)
Casual	22 (119)	37 (387)	8 (198)	30 (105)
Prostitute	100 (24)	100 (36)	100 (4)	100 (4)

n = total number of partnerships of this type.

[a] In Yaoundé the categories "girlfriend" and "fiancée" were not distinguished.

Table 3.6. *Estimates of Rate of Sex Work Contact in Each of the Four Cities*

	Cotonou	Yaoundé	Kisumu	Ndola
From survey of men				
% men with contacts in the last year	4	12	3	6
Contacts per 1000 men per year	130–160	1800–2750	490–540	1050–1900
From survey of sex workers				
Client contacts per 1000 city-resident men per year	3360	1700	960	3330

girlfriends and none were described as fiancées. Using the definition in Box 3.2 HIV prevalence in "clients" and other men was similar in Cotonou and Kisumu, but there was some indication that it was higher in "clients" in Yaoundé and Ndola ($P = 0.07$ and $P = 0.09$, respectively). Similarly syphilis was not significantly higher among "clients" than other men except in Yaoundé ($P < 0.01$). Between 29 and 34 percent of "clients" had other non-spousal partners aged less than 20.

Table 3.6 shows estimates of the extent of contact with sex workers according to the male population data and the survey of sex workers. Apart from Yaoundé there are major discrepancies between the two sets of figures with estimates based on men being much lower. The discrepancy in Cotonou is particularly great.

3.5.2.3 Discussion
Defining contact with sex workers in the last year using the characteristics of non-spousal data was not straightforward. Exchange of money did not appear to be a

useful criterion for defining sex work contact, and other characteristics of the partners of the male informants had large proportions of missing data. The "clients" identified that using the definition did not have consistently higher prevalence of HIV or syphilis than other men, and this persisted after excluding those contacts in which condoms were used. This suggests that using the characteristics of the relationship to define sex work leads to misclassification and that probing the respondent on whether any of his partners might be considered to be sex workers might be more sensitive and specific. However, a major problem with this latter approach is that sex work is not easy to distinguish in an African context and both partners might regard the relationship as something else. Further work needs to be done to develop probing questions on contacts with sex workers for future questionnaires.

Large discrepancies were found between the extent of contact with sex workers estimated from reports by men compared to sex workers. While some of this could be due to problems with the definition of contact with sex workers and the crude assumptions on which the calculations are based, the discrepancies are large enough to merit consideration. Some of the discrepancy could be because clients of the sex workers might be from other core-groups such as the bar owners, the military or truck drivers and that these groups would not be included in the household survey. Another possible explanation is bias introduced by non-participation in the surveys of the male population: it is possible that the substantial proportions of men not interviewed (most of whom were "not found" rather than refusals) had more contact with sex workers. However, the city with the largest discrepancy, Cotonou, had a high response rate for men (95 percent) so this is unlikely to be an explanation there. In conclusion, allowing for the crudeness of the figures calculated, the triangulation still suggests that men are not reporting sexual partners who are sex workers or reporting them as partners without the label "sex worker." This is likely to greatly bias surveys in which this type of data is collected.

3.5.3 Investigating the causes of the disparity in HIV prevalence between young men and young women

It has been noted in several areas in sub-Saharan Africa that the HIV prevalence in women is high within the first few years of sexual activity, whereas that in men rises more slowly (Kwesigabo et al. 1996; Fontanet et al. 1998; Fylkesnes et al. 1998; Boerma et al. 1999). While this could be an artifact due to failure to include, through absence or refusal, young men with higher rates of HIV seropositivity, the consistency of the finding and the magnitude of the difference makes this unlikely as a full explanation.

Women may have higher HIV prevalence then men because they are more exposed to infected partners and/or because they are at higher risk of acquiring HIV infection from an infected partner. There is some evidence that HIV transmission from men to women is more efficient than from women to men (Mastro and de Vincenzi 1996). Several studies in discordant couples in Africa and elsewhere have found higher seroconversion rates in the initially seronegative female partners of male index cases, than in the initially seronegative male partners of female index cases (Hira et al. 1990;

Padian et al. 1997; Carpenter et al. 1999; Senkoro et al. 2000), though other studies have found similar seroconversion rates for men and women in HIV discordant partnerships (de Vincenzi 1994; Serwadda et al. 1995; Fideli et al. 2000; Quinn et al. 2000). In areas of high STD prevalence it has been suggested that any difference in male to female and female to male HIV transmission probabilities may be counterbalanced by the presence of other STDs and higher co-factor effects in female to male transmission (Vernazza et al. 1999). Comparison of transmission is further complicated by likely variation in transmission probability over the course of the infection, and the fact that discordant couples are a selected group in which transmission has not occurred in the earliest stages of infection (Mastro and de Vincenzi 1996).

Sexual network data can be used to investigate the other potential explanation for the higher HIV prevalence in women than in men—that they are more exposed to infected partners. The risk of exposure to an infected partner at a young age depends on the age at sexual debut, the number of partners, and the likelihood that those partners are infected. This will depend on the type of partnership, the age of the partner, and the partner's risk behavior. We analyzed data from the two high prevalence sites, Kisumu and Ndola, to explore these factors and to assess the extent to which differences in risk of exposure to an infected partner can explain the disparity in HIV prevalence between young men and young women (Glynn et al. 2001).

3.5.3.1 Methods used in the analyses

The distribution of the age at sexual debut, the number of lifetime partners, and the proportions married at each age were compared between men and women. The risk of HIV within marriage for women was examined in relation to the age difference from their husband and by whether they were virgins at the time of marriage. Virginity at the time of marriage was not asked directly in the questionnaire and those who had sexual intercourse with their future spouse before marriage may or may not have counted them as premarital partners. For this analysis we defined virgins at marriage as *either* those with no declared premarital partners *or* those with one declared premarital partner *and* the same age at sexual debut as at marriage.

Details for non-marital partnerships used the information collected on all sexual partnerships (up to eight) during the previous 12 months. Results were analyzed to explore the proportion of young women and young men with older partners and the proportion of older men with young female partners but the results could not be reconciled.

HIV prevalence increases with age and is higher in married individuals than those who are unmarried. To see whether the age difference in non-marital partnerships explained the differences seen in HIV prevalence, the age distribution, and marital status of declared partners in the last 12 months were used to estimate the probability of infection in the partners of unmarried men and women under 20. This was done in three different ways.

1. We used the HIV prevalence of men who reported that they had had sex with unmarried women under 20 (in the last 12 months), and the HIV prevalence of

women who reported that they had had sex with unmarried men under 20 (in the last 12 months). These were calculated both crudely and after weighting by the number of partners in that category. The calculations were also repeated including those with partners with unknown age and marital status.

2. The age distribution of the partners of individuals who had had only one lifetime partner was compared with the age–sex–marital status specific HIV prevalence in the population to estimate the probability of HIV infection in the partners. (These partner ages were only available if the partner was seen in the last 12 months.)

3. To estimate the *maximum* probability of HIV infection in male partners the partnership histories of each woman were examined. Since HIV seropositivity increases with age and is higher in married men, the maximum probability of HIV infection was estimated from the prevalence of HIV by age of men in the population, using the age of the oldest partner and taking the age-specific prevalence for married men if any of the woman's partners were married. Partners under 15 years were assumed to be HIV negative. For men the *minimum* probability of HIV infection in a partner was calculated similarly, using the age of their youngest partner and the prevalence for unmarried women if any of the partners were unmarried.

Finally, the relative risk of HIV between women and men was compared directly in a multivariate logistic regression model, allowing for marriage, number of partners, age at sexual debut, and the presence of STDs, to assess the extent to which measured differences in behavior and STDs could explain the differences in HIV prevalence seen. The sensitivity of the results to the accuracy of partnership histories was explored by doubling or tripling the number of partners for the women, and also by excluding number of partners from the model.

3.5.3.2 *Outline of results*
Results are presented in detail elsewhere (Glynn et al. 2001). In both sites age at sexual debut was similar for men and women, and men declared many more partners than did women, so these factors did not explain the disparity in HIV prevalence. Women married at a younger age than men and marriage was a risk factor for HIV, but this did not explain the male–female discrepancy in HIV prevalence since differences in HIV prevalence between men and women were seen in both married and unmarried individuals. HIV prevalence was lower in women with a small age difference from their husbands and in those who were virgins at marriage.

Young men had very few older partners whereas about one fifth of unmarried women under 20 with non-marital partners in the last 12 months had had at least one partner over 24. The estimates of the HIV prevalence in the partners suggested that the probability of a partner being infected is probably similar for the young single men and women in these two sites. Since men had more partners their risk of having an infected partner was actually higher than that for the women.

The direct comparison of the risk of HIV between men and women showed a greatly increased risk of HIV in young women compared with young men, having

80 *Michael Caraël et al.*

controlled for partnership factors and STDs. The results suggest that the different transmission probabilities between men and women are a crucial factor in driving the distribution of HIV.

3.5.3.3 Discussion

The analyses rely on comparing the information provided by young men and young women. Any inaccuracies in those data, and any bias in the responses, particularly if different for men and women, will bias the results. There were some reasons for questioning the validity of the partnership data. Very few women declared unmarried male partners under 20, but the information from the unmarried men under 20 suggests that there should have been many more. A high proportion of women, 11–18 percent, (and 8–9 percent of men) who denied ever having been sexually active were infected with HIV and other STDs. The HIV prevalence in young unmarried women with one lifetime partner was implausibly high given the HIV prevalence in men in the population and the fact that the efficiency of transmission of HIV is less than 100 percent.

Further evidence comes from data on married couples who were both seen in the study. In Kisumu, of twenty-two women who claimed one lifetime partner and had an HIV negative husband, two were HIV positive. In Ndola six of seventy-one such women with HIV-negative husbands were HIV positive. (Equivalent figures for men were one of four in Kisumu and one of ten in Ndola.) This suggests that women under report total number of partners and high risk partners.

The three different methods used to estimate the HIV prevalence in partners gave similar results, though some were based on small numbers. Many men declared unmarried female partners under 20, and the HIV prevalence in these men is probably a reasonable estimate of the average HIV prevalence in the partners of the young women. It relies on appropriate sampling of the men, the accuracy of their partnership histories, and their HIV status. It may underestimate the HIV prevalence if there is a small highly active "core group" of men with high HIV prevalence who are likely to be missed in a general population sample. This method did not work well for estimating the HIV prevalence in female partners of young men because few women declared young male partners, giving unstable and probably biased results.

The best estimate of HIV prevalence in the partners of the men is probably that based on the third method. Because the analysis was attempting to explain discrepancies in male and female HIV prevalence as far as possible, this measure was designed to estimate a minimum HIV prevalence (for comparison with a maximum for the women). If an average estimate were required rather than a minimum, the method could be adapted by using, for example, the average age of the partners or by considering all partnerships.

The use of different methods to obtain estimates of HIV prevalence for the partners of the men and of the women may have some advantages. Both preferred methods rely on the men's partnership histories, so their comparison avoids any differences in reporting bias between men and women. The use of more than one method for both men and women helps to check the results.

3.6 SUMMARY

The questionnaire was designed to overcome weaknesses in that used in earlier surveys (GPA/WHO), in particular the lack of detail on the characteristics of regular as well as casual partnerships (Cleland et al. 1995). The addition of a biological component, measuring HIV and other STIs, allows more detailed analysis of the dynamics and determinants of the HIV epidemic.

The new questionnaire was feasible for use in a field survey by interviewers without specific skills except for those provided by 5 days of training. Despite the invasive nature of some of the questions it was well accepted by the respondents. To some extent it measured what it was supposed to measure: within each site the expected relationships were found between different measures of sexual behavior, and between these measures and STIs, including HIV. We are, however, aware of various limitations. We have already seen that some questions had poor response rates, and there was a suggestion of questionnaire—or interviewer—fatigue. There is also evidence of under-reporting of sexual partners, particularly by women, and of under-reporting of commercial sex contacts by men. In all sites some men and women who denied sexual activity had STIs and in Kisumu and Ndola the HIV prevalence in women with one declared lifetime partner was implausibly high. In all sites men reported many more partners than did women, and this discrepancy is probably greater than can easily be explained by postulating partnerships outside the survey population (Buvé et al. 2001). Because most of the questions on sexual behavior were asked in terms of identified partners and partnerships, it is quite possible that short encounters, particularly coercive and violent sex, may not have been mentioned, particularly by women. These may need to be asked about specifically, but this requires attention to the action that will be given if violence is uncovered. A follow-up qualitative study in Kisumu suggests that women are under-reporting their sexual partnerships and that sexual coercion, sometimes at an early age, is not uncommon (Njue 1999). This emphasizes the continuing need for linked qualitative studies to allow triangulation with survey results.

The questionnaire is already quite long, at least for those with multiple partners, but inevitably there are more questions that would be useful to add. Some points need further clarification. For example, it is important to be able to distinguish whether the number of premarital partners given includes the spouse; to know specifically about virginity at the time of marriage; to ask specifically about the characteristics of the first sexual partner, and the circumstances of the first relationship; to ask specifically about concurrency. Individuals may have difficulties recalling dates and durations of relationships, but are likely to know whether overlap occurred. More needs to be done to define contact with a FSW, perhaps including specific probing questions, and to test the suggested definition (Box 3.2). For further exploring the vulnerability of young women, questions on menarche should be included.

The information collected by this study has been used for a number of analyses other than those described here, including detailed studies of risk factors for HIV and other STIs, sexual behavior, and relationships with marriage. The study was designed to allow comparison of biological and behavioral risk factors for HIV between the study sites. This aspect was used, for example, in comparing concurrency indices between sites. Because a common methodology was used in each city, the design also allows immediate testing of hypotheses raised in one site in another setting. For example, the finding that the higher HIV prevalence in young women than in young men seems to depend more on different susceptibilities to HIV than on different risks of encountering HIV infected partners, is made more compelling by the parallel results in Kisumu and Ndola.

The questionnaire has also been used in other studies (e.g. in Senegal, Burkina Faso, and South Africa) with and without the biological component. It is freely available (www.unaids.org) and continued use of this standardized instrument should aid further comparative studies and allow monitoring of changes over time.

References

Alary, M., Lowndes, C. et al. (1999). "Male clients of prostitutes in Benin: STD prevalence and associated risk factors," *13th Meeting of the International Society for Sexually Transmitted Diseases Research,* Denver (Abstract #050).

Anderson, R., May, R. et al. (1991). "The spread of HIV-1 in Africa: Sexual contact patterns and the predicted demographic impact of AIDS," *Nature,* 352: 581–9.

Boerma, J., Urassa, M. et al. (1999). "Spread of HIV infection in a rural area of Tanzania," *AIDS* 13: 1233–40.

Buvé, A., Carael, M. et al. (2001). "Multicentre study on factors determining differences in rate of spread of HIV in sub-Saharan Africa: Methods and prevalence of HIV infection," *AIDS,* 15(Suppl 4): S5–14.

—— Caraël, M. et al. (1995). "Variations in HIV prevalence between urban areas in sub-Saharan Africa: Do we understand them?" *AIDS,* 9(Suppl A): S103–9.

—— Lagarde, E. et al. (2001). "Interpreting sexual behavior data: Validity issues in the multicentre study on factors determining the differential spread of HIV in four African cities," *AIDS,* 15(Suppl 4): S117–26.

Carael, M., Cleland, J. et al. (1991). "Overview and selected findings of sexual behaviour surveys. [Review]," *AIDS,* 5(Suppl 1): S65–74.

Carpenter, L., Kamali, A. et al. (1999). "Rates of HIV-1 transmission within marriage in rural Uganda in relation to the HIV serostatus of the partners," *AIDS,* 13: 1083–9.

Cleland, J., Ferry, B. et al. (1995). "Sexual behavior and AIDS in the developing world." In J. Cleland and B. Ferry (eds.), London: Taylor and Francis, pp. 208–31.

de Vincenzi, I. (1994). "A longitudinal study of human immunodeficiency virus transmission by heterosexual partners. European study group on heterosexual transmission of HIV. *Engl J Med,* 331: 341–6.

Fideli, U., Allen, S. et al. (2000). "*Virological determinants of heterosexual transmission in Africa,*" 7th Conference on Retroviruses and Opportunistic Infections, Foundation for Retrovirology and Human Health (Abstract 194).

Fontanet, A., Messele, T. et al. (1998). "Age- and sex-specific HIV-1 prevalence in the urban community setting of Addis Ababa, Ethiopia." *AIDS,* 12: 315–22.

Fylkesnes, K., Ndhlovu, Z. et al. (1998). "Studying dynamics of the HIV epidemic: Population-based data compared with sentinel surveillance in Zambia." *AIDS*, 12: 1227–34.

Garnett, G. and Johnson, A. (1997). "Coining a new term in epidemiology: Concurrency and HIV," *AIDS*, 11: 681–3.

Ghani, A. C., Swinton, J. et al. (1997). "The role of sexual partnership networks in the epidemiology of gonorrhea," *Sex Transm Dis*, 24(1): 45–56.

Global Programme on AIDS (WHO/GPA 1994). *Evaluation of a National AIDS Programme: A Methods Package*. Geneva: World Health Organization.

Glynn, J. R., Caraël, M. et al. (2001). "Why do young women have a much higher prevalence of HIV than young men? A study in Kisumu, Kenya and Ndola, Zambia." *AIDS*, 15(Suppl 4): S51–60.

Hira, S., Nkowane, B. et al. (1990). "Epidemiology of human immunodeficiency virus in families in Lusaka, Zambia," *J AIDS*, 3(1): 83–6.

Hudson, C. (1993). "Concurrent partners and the results of the Uganda Rakai project [letter]." *AIDS*, 7: 236–43.

Hudson, C. (1996). "AIDS in rural Africa: A paradigm for HIV-1 prevention," *Int J STD and AIDS*, 7: 236–43.

Huygens, P. and Caraël, M. (1998). Multicentre study on determinants of differences in HIV prevalence: Anthropological Assessment. Geneva, UNAIDS/PSR Research Report.

Kretzschmar, M. and Morris, M. (1996). "Measures of concurrency in networks and the spread of infectious disease." *Math Biosc*, 133: 165–95.

Kwesigabo, G., Killewo, J. et al. (1996). "Sentinel surveillance and cross sectional survey on HIV infection prevalence: A comparative study," *East African Med J*, 73: 198–302.

Lagarde, E., Auvert, B. et al. (2001). "Concurrent sexual partnerships and HIV prevalence in five urban communities of sub-Saharan Africa," *AIDS*, 15: 877–84.

Mastro, T. and de Vincenzi, I. (1996). "Probabilities of sexual HIV-1 transmission," *AIDS*, 10(Suppl A): S75–82.

Mehret, M., Mertens, T et al. (1996). "Baseline for the evaluation of an AIDS programme using prevention indicators: A case study in Ethiopia." *Bull WHO*, 74: 509–16.

Mertens, T. and Caraël, M. (1997). "Evaluation of HIV/STD prevention, care and support: An update on WHO's approaches," *AIDS Educ Prev*, 9: 133–45.

—— —— et al. (1994). "Prevention indicators for evaluating the progress of National AIDS Intervention Programmes," *AIDS*, 8: 1359–69.

Mills, S., Saidel, T. et al. (1998). "HIV risk behavioral surveillance: A methodology for monitoring behavioral trends," *AIDS*, 12(Suppl 2): S37–46.

Morison, L., Weiss, H. et al. (2001). "Commercial sex and the spread of HIV in four cities in sub-Saharan Africa," *AIDS*, 15(Suppl 4): S61–9.

Morris, M. (1997). "Sexual networks and HIV," *AIDS*, 11(Suppl A): S209–16.

—— and Kretzschmar, M. (1997). "Concurrent partnerships and the spread of HIV," *AIDS*, 11: 641–8.

——, Podhisita, C. et al. (1996). "Bridge populations in the spread of HIV/AIDS in Thailand," *AIDS*, 11: 1265–71.

Njue, C. (1999). "Study on youth sexual behaviour. Additional qualitative studies in Kisumu: The Kenya site for the multi-centre study on factors determining the differential spread of HIV infection in African Towns," Unpublished report for UNAIDS.

Padian, N., Shiboski, S. et al. (1997). "Heterosexual transmission of human immunodeficiency virus (HIV) in northern California: Results from a ten year study," *Am J Epidemiol*, 146: 350–7.

Pickering, H., Todd, J. et al. (1992). "Prostitutes and their clients: A Gambian survey," *Social Sci Med*, 341: 75–88.

Quinn, T., Wawer, M. et al. (2000). "Viral load and heterosexual transmission of human immunodeficiency virus type 1," *N Engl J Med*, 342: 921–9.

Senkoro, K., Boerma, J. et al. (2000). "HIV incidence and HIV-associated mortality in a cohort of factory workers and their spouses in Tanzania, 1991 through 1996," *J AIDS*, 23: 194–202.

Serwadda, D., Gray, R. et al. (1995). "The social dynamics of HIV transmission as reflected through discordant couples in rural Uganda," *AIDS*, 9: 745–50.

UNAIDS (1998). "Looking deeper into the HIV epidemic. A questionnaire for tracing sexual networks." *UNAIDS Best Practice Collection*, UNAIDS/98.27.

Vernazza, P., Eron, J. et al. (1999). "Sexual transmission of HIV: Infectiousness and prevention," *AIDS*, 13: 155–66.

Watts, C. H. and May, R. M. (1992). "The influence of concurrent partnerships on the dynamics of HIV/AIDS," *Math Biosc*, 108: 89–104.

PART II

PARTIAL NETWORK DESIGNS

4

Network Dynamism: History and Lessons of the Colorado Springs Study

JOHN J. POTTERAT, DONALD E. WOODHOUSE, STEPHEN Q.
MUTH, RICHARD B. ROTHENBERG, WILLIAM W. DARROW,
ALDEN S. KLOVDAHL, AND JOHN B. MUTH

> Never underestimate the complexity of social network research
> Alden Klovdahl

4.1 INTRODUCTION

This endeavor, begun in the autumn of 1987, was the first prospective study of the influence of network structure on the propagation of infectious disease. Funded by the Centers for Disease Control and Prevention (CDC) to explore the dynamics of human immunodeficiency virus (HIV) transmission in heterosexual populations, the project was intended to build on the work of Klovdahl who, a few years earlier, proposed application of the social network paradigm to infectious disease epidemiology (Klovdahl 1985).

In the mid-1980s the CDC channeled part of its investigative energies to assess the magnitude and direction of the HIV epidemic in heterosexual populations (Centers for Disease Control and Prevention 1987). Among its first priorities was determining HIV prevalence and associated risk factors in prostitute women; of the eight participating sites in the United States (Centers for Disease Control and Prevention 1987; Khabbaz et al. 1990), Colorado Springs was selected because of its long-term public health partnership with prostitute women (Potterat et al. 1979; Potterat et al. 1985; Potterat et al. 1999) and because it was believed to represent "Middle America."

The following contributors, in alphabetical order, assisted in the design of the behavior questionnaire: Sabine Bartholomeyczik, Jackie Boles, Judith Cohen, William Darrow, Kirk Elifson, John Gagnon, Rima Khabbaz, Alden Klovdahl, Stephen Muth, Lynn Plummer, John Potterat, Claire Sterk, Donald Woodhouse, and Constance Wofsy. We thank the principal interviewers: Lynn Plummer, John Potterat, Helen Zimmerman-Rogers, Donald Woodhouse, and Helen Zimmerman. Special thanks to Tammy Maldonado for extraordinary patience and dedication in the completion of the tedious de-duplication routines; to Nancy Brace for useful discussions; to Frank Judson, MD for Institutional Review Board assistance; and to the United States Air Force Academy for providing access to an Evans & Sutherland graphics workstation. Data collection instruments, codebooks, and data sets are available from the authors in Colorado Springs (sqmuth@earthlink.net or jjpotterat@earthlink.net).

This study, conducted during 1986–7, found that HIV infection in prostitute women was associated with injecting drug use (IDU) and, to a lesser extent, with unprotected vaginal intercourse (Centers for Disease Control and Prevention 1987). At completion its principal investigator, William Darrow, invited three sites to participate in a joint project to elucidate mechanisms of HIV incidence in populations of men and women participating in prostitution and/or IDU. Because one of us doubted HIV's ability to significantly propagate in non-injecting heterosexual populations (Potterat et al. 1986; Potterat 1987; Potterat et al. 1987), Darrow suggested exploring the larger social networks of heterosexuals perceived to be at high risk for HIV infection in Colorado Springs. Not only had he long been interested in the social context of sexually transmitted disease (STD) transmission (Darrow et al. 1999), as had the Colorado Springs staff (Rothenberg 1983; Potterat et al. 1985), but he and Klovdahl had corresponded in the early 1980s about the potential usefulness of a social network approach to understanding the "Patient Zero" outbreak (Auerbach et al. 1984; Klovdahl 1985). The hope was that this paradigm, newly imported from the social sciences, might provide insights into the dynamics of HIV propagation.

4.2 STUDY PRELIMINARIES

4.2.1 *The name of the game is names*

For completeness, description of social networks (in contrast to personal networks) requires precise identification of actors by name (Klovdahl 1989). Given the general concern for confidentiality engendered by the HIV epidemic and considering that the contemplated study required asking for such data in the absence of the customary stimulus (presence of communicable disease), initial concern focused on feasibility. Although Colorado Springs staff had extensive experience with contact tracing for both STD and HIV infections—and had, indeed, used an implicit network approach to elucidate STD patterns (Potterat et al. 1985)—no staff member had ever attempted to elicit the names and locating information for "contacts" of persons who were not known to be infected. Because of time-honored association with elusive and disenfranchised populations at risk for STD/HIV in Colorado Springs and because HIV/AIDS reporting was universal and actively monitored (Potterat et al. 1993), it was concluded that such a site would be a suitable testing ground. In addition, both the size and confined geography of Colorado Springs made it an attractive choice. Lastly, low HIV prevalence among local heterosexuals made it appear an ideal population in which to observe transmission over time; hence, of the three sites invited to continue participation with CDC in prostitution settings, only Colorado Springs was invited to use a formal network approach.

4.2.2 *Expert assistance*

In 1987, the Colorado Springs STD/HIV staff consisted of four local health department contact tracers and clerical support. None had advanced academic qualifications. None was familiar with survey or sample design and none knew that social network analysis existed. None was familiar with computer databases; indeed, the STD/HIV program did not own a computer. From the beginning it was understood that outside expertise would be needed to conceptualize the study; to design data collection instruments; to enter, collate, and analyze network data; and to recommend computer equipment and software. In the autumn of 1987, the resources to obtain this assistance materialized as a cooperative agreement between the Health Department in Colorado Springs and the AIDS Program at the CDC in Atlanta; Darrow, chief of the AIDS Behavioral Branch, was assigned as project officer.

4.3 SAMPLE

4.3.1 *Study site and enrollment criteria*

Colorado Springs is a geographically well-bounded middle size community near the center of the United States. Its metropolitan area, located 100 km south of Denver, comprised nearly 400,000 persons in 1990, of whom about 70 percent resided in the city and 30 percent in sparsely populated rural areas. Approximately 80 percent of its residents were White, 9 percent Latino, 7 percent African-American (AA), and the remainder, "Other." About 32,000 were active duty military personnel assigned to four Army and Air Force installations. Members of heterosexual populations perceived, at the time, to be at high risk of HIV transmission were targeted for recruitment: prostitute women, IDUs, and their respective partners.

Four criteria to establish eligibility for enrollment were initially used. That is, heterosexual or bisexual persons at least 18 years of age needed to have had a history, during the 12 months preceding interview, of:

1. Exchanging sex for money or drugs;
2. Sex (paying or nonpaying) with a prostitute;
3. Injection of illicit drugs; or
4. Sex with IDU.

4.3.2 *Sampling strategies and informed consent*

The problem of "sampling" prostitute women presented no conceptual difficulties: the number of such women and of their nonpaying partners (e.g. pimps, boyfriends, etc.) was known to be small enough to attempt recruiting the whole population. About 100–120 prostitutes (Potterat et al. 1990) and about thirty pimps were estimated to be in the Colorado Springs area in a given year. Parenthetically, during the study's 40-month *enrollment* period, 217 different prostitutes were actually observed. Contact tracers had developed trusting relationships with members of the local prostitution scene since 1970 (Potterat et al. 1979, 1999) through the STD clinic and through regular outreach to areas frequented by prostitutes (Centers for Disease Control and Prevention 1992). Goals of these outreach efforts included contact tracing, condom distribution, safer sex advice, bleach distribution to encourage sterilization of needles, and referral to social and medical services (Plummer et al. 1996).

As of 1987, estimates of the number of IDU in Colorado Springs were unavailable and the STD/HIV staff had had only modest experience with such populations. The same was true for paying partners of prostitutes. Sampling in these two populations presented major conceptual difficulties. Klovdahl, familiar with the theoretical issues of network sampling, initially considered using approaches based on Frank's work (Frank 1978); exploring various forms of purposive sampling (Johnson 1990); and link-tracing sampling, including his own Random Walk approach (Klovdahl 1989). In the end, site-based recruiting, coupled with link-tracing, was used. The strategy was to enroll as many of the IDU population through the methadone clinic and through observed network links (e.g. IDU nominated by respondents), based on the optimistic guess that it would not be unmanageably large. Finally, as many paying partners of prostitutes as possible were to be recruited from health department STD/HIV testing sites; from outreach efforts in places known to be frequented by such persons, and from lists of paying partners identified by prostitute women in the network section of the survey instrument. Enrollment was intended to be continuous for 60 months, with baseline respondents being interviewed at yearly follow-up intervals for up to 5 years.

Because of the large military populations in Colorado Springs and their previous significance for both STD transmission and prostitution (Woodhouse et al. 1985), efforts were made to recruit from military clinics. Regrettably, the previously cordial working relationship between health department and military public health workers was severely strained by publication, in the spring of 1987, of a letter perceived by the military as reflecting adversely on their professional competence (Potterat et al. 1987). Although reconciliation efforts were attempted in the summer of 1987, they proved futile until 1991, by which time recruitment of new respondents was ending. Thus, our plan to draw eligible respondents from the entire community was affected—to what extent is unknown—by inability to tap military venues.

The study design and survey instruments were approved by the Institutional Review Board (IRB) of the University of Colorado Health Sciences Center. Respondents were asked to sign a consent form, which was also verbally explained in plain English. This form included a statement of the research purpose; discussion of potential risks and benefits; a statement about confidentiality of records; details about whom to contact for complaints or information; a statement emphasizing the voluntary nature of participation and the revocable nature of consent. Participants were recruited from health department STD, HIV, and substance abuse clinics, where patients were routinely queried for eligibility; from vice-squad referrals; street outreach; and from lists of frequently named respondents.

4.4 DATA COLLECTION

The study's aim was to prospectively test the basic proposition that "the structure of a network has consequences for its individual members and for the network as a whole over and above the effects of characteristics and behaviour of the individuals involved" (Klovdahl et al. 1994) in the transmission of AIDS. Accomplishing this aim required collection of both behavioral and network data. Accordingly, survey instruments comprised two parts: a behavior- and a network-oriented questionnaire. The behavioral questionnaire was based on existing instruments developed primarily by researchers at Georgia State University; the latter, chiefly by Klovdahl of the Australian National University.

4.4.1 Behavioral questionnaire

This section, which consumed approximately one-half hour, sought to obtain sociodemographic data (16 variables) and a brief STD/HIV medical and risk history, including contraceptive and condom use (15 variables). It also included a detailed probe of illicit drug use (68 variables), with especial focus on IDU behavior and by a similar probe of the respondent's sexual history (twenty-one variables), with especial focus on anal sex. While the main period of interest was the preceding 12 months, some questions about sexual and drug behaviors sought information covering the previous 5 years. Replies to questions in these subsections, along with a brief set of Knowledge, Attitudes, Beliefs (KAB) questions (sixteen variables), were also used as a springboard to counsel the respondent about safer behaviors. Therefore, *intervention was a significant aspect of interaction with respondents*; it included safer behaviors educational messages, referral to drug rehabilitation, and free condom distribution (Centers for Disease Control and Prevention 1992; Klovdahl et al. 1994). Lastly, the respondent was asked to estimate the number of social, sex, and drug partners during the 6 months preceding interview. These three additional questions were intended to measure the accuracy of partner estimates versus partner enumeration, which forms the core of the next section.

4.4.2 Network questionnaire

This section, designed in December of 1987, required approximately 1 h to complete. Its purpose was to elicit the names of the respondent's social, sexual, illicit drug, and injecting drug partners for the prior 6 months. Identifying social partners permits delineation of the respondent's *social* network, while identifying sexual and drug partners allows construction of their *risk* network. Approximately thirty-six variables about each named partner were included. Parenthetically, to prevent interview fatigue leading to an artifactual curtailing of partner listings, only the partner's first name and first initial of last name were requested at first; when the list was considered "complete" details about each partner were solicited subsequently. Questions focused on partner demographics (e.g. age, ethnicity, gender, occupation), locating information (e.g. last name, nickname, address, telephone), relationship to respondent (e.g. neighbor, co-worker, relative), frequency and strength of relationship (on a scale of 1–10), and nature of relationship (e.g. detail on: sexual exposures and practices, including condom use; and frequency and kinds of drug use practices). These questions comprised twenty-eight variables (see Appendix).

The rationale for soliciting the names of social and risk partners was presented to respondents as follows:

We are concerned with preventing the spread of diseases such as AIDS virus infection, and also with preventing the spread of other diseases spread by close or intimate personal contact. For our purposes, 'close personal contact' includes:

1. sharing meals (regularly or periodically)
2. sharing living quarters
3. sharing clothes or other personal possessions
4. sexual contact
5. using drugs or getting high together.

This broad definition of personal relationships was deliberate and based on four considerations: (*a*) emphasizing to respondents that our interest was disease prevention, not illicit or illegal activities, (*b*) understanding the transmission context of a broad range of infectious agents, not just HIV, (*c*) observing the (de)evolution of, say, purely social to risky relationships and vice-versa, and (*d*) observing the larger social context in which risky relationships were embedded (Klovdahl et al. 1994). We were also aware that had our name generator been more narrowly focused, our ability to observe connected regions of the overall social network might have been impaired if risky relationships were sparsely distributed in the population.

At the end of this section, up to sixteen named partners were arrayed in a triangular matrix and respondents were asked to describe three relationships between them (e.g. does person A know, have sex with, or do drugs with, person B?), and to list one close associate for each listed partner (a concept borrowed from syphilis epidemiology, "cluster interviewing"). Lastly, respondents who were partners of prostitute women were asked an additional fifteen questions designed to probe their sexual preferences and practices with prostitutes, as well as their motivation for soliciting them.

4.4.3. Blood testing and remuneration

Respondents were asked to provide a blood specimen (30 ml) for HIV, syphilis, hepatitis-B, and Human T-Lymphotropic Virus (HTLV) testing at baseline and at follow-up interview; they were informed that specimens would be stored for possible future testing, in case reliable tests for associated STD or bloodborne infections (e.g. herpes-I, II; hepatitis-C) became available.

No remuneration was offered during the first 2 years of the study, because we did not think it was necessary and because we felt that it might bias enrollment. By 1990 we had learned, from studies conducted elsewhere, that paying participants was common and that such recompense significantly biased neither participant selection nor data validity. Importantly, a major operational challenge consisted of locating our frequently peripatetic respondents for follow-up interviews; we reasoned that remuneration would stimulate—and it did!—respondents to seek us out at yearly intervals. Thus, starting with Year-III interviews, respondents were paid a graduated honorarium of US$15 for the initial, $25 for the second, and $35 for subsequent, interviews.

4.4.4 Follow-up interviews

To assess the potential influence of changes in network configuration over time, respondents were to be interviewed at yearly intervals for up to 5 years. Survey length was similar to that of the baseline instrument but differed slightly in content. Questions were designed to capture changes during the previous 12 months in the respondent's demographics (e.g. current address, mobility, occupation); in sexual and reproductive health; and in HIV risk behaviors. Repeat of the network survey (same as B above) focused on eliciting network partners during the previous 6 months. No data from a previous respondent interview was included in the same respondent's follow-up interview(s) or questionnaire(s); responses between first and follow-up interviews were compared subsequently.

Survey instruments were designed during the first 2 months of 1988, pilot tested on ten participants during March, and approved by the IRB in April 1988. Year-I interviews started on 1 May 1988 and were completed 30 April 1989. All interviews were conducted face-to-face at a site of the respondent's choosing: at the health department, at home, in a car, at some outdoor location, or in jail. Completion of all items required, on average, 1.5 h (range 1–2.5 h). No tape recording or video equipment was used.

4.5 FIELD EXPERIENCES

4.5.1 Staff, training, and costs

The study staff consisted of 3.5 full-time equivalent positions: a full-time project manager/interviewer, three part-time interviewers, a full-time data entry clerk, and a part-time data manager. The interviewers were STD/HIV contact tracers with a mean age of 41 years (sd: 9.6) and with a mean of 8.8 years (sd: 6.8) of interviewing experience. The cost of this 5-year project was $786,442. Because the interviewers were seasoned STD/HIV contact tracers, little training beyond familiarization with the new data instruments was required. It is our opinion that STD/HIV contact interviewing and contact tracing experience is crucial for network studies that explore sensitive personal behaviors and their social context. Such experience fosters interviewer confidence, encourages use of non-apologetic, positively phrased questions, and the use of techniques of suggestion that improve recall (Potterat et al. 1991).

4.5.2 Mid-course corrections

Because we had earned the trust of prostitute women over time, recruitment efforts initially focused on them. As the number of enrollable local prostitutes diminished during the second year (because already enrolled and because of our community's moderate prostitute turn-over rate), greater emphasis was placed on recruiting non-prostitute IDU, paying customers of prostitutes, and "cross-links" (Klovdahl 1989). The latter were persons who were named by more than one respondent (Klovdahl et al. 1977); they were preferentially targeted for interview to enhance the probability of observing connections between the ostensibly disparate subpopulations we sought to enroll.

The small number of IDU ($n = 65$) attending our health department methadone clinic in 1987 provided modest opportunities to enroll new participants. In addition, clinic IDU were usually in the process of leaving drug networks, and were primarily addicted to heroin. To enroll IDU not currently in treatment or who were injecting drugs other than heroin—principally amphetamines—we made special efforts to recruit, through outreach and respondent referral, non-prostitute IDU in Year II. In addition, a separate category for crack use was made to capture this new form of cocaine ingestion.

By spring of 1990, availability of polymerase chain reaction (PCR) technology and refinement of lymphocyte enumeration techniques induced us to collect blood specimens specifically intended for such testing. Lastly, testing of blood samples for antibody to HTLV was discontinued at the end of the first year because no positives were identified.

4.5.3 Ethical and legal considerations

The exigencies of collecting blood specimens for HIV testing and of gathering sensitive personal behavior data linked to personal identifiers presented challenging ethical, legal, and operational questions. We have detailed these issues elsewhere (Klovdahl 1995; Woodhouse et al. 1995). In brief, we were concerned that confidential—as opposed to anonymous—HIV testing might discourage potential participants, with implications for recruitment strategies and sampling assessments. We did not use anonymous, or "blinded" specimen testing, because mapping the precise location of HIV-positive persons in network structures was considered crucial, because we believed that knowing HIV status would be more beneficial than harmful to the respondents themselves, and because anonymous testing was not permitted in Colorado. Participants were informed that positive results would be reported by name to health authorities and that risk partners would require notification. Because participants could not be given the option not to know their results, this presented a potential clash with legal requirements that subjects be able to "withdraw" from the study at any time. At no time did any participant elect to withdraw from the study.

Previous experience indicated that at least some prostitute women in Colorado Springs were less than 18 years old. Our review of Colorado law, which permits minors to consent to diagnosis, treatment, and follow-up for sexually transmissible disease, substance abuse, or birth control, led us to conclude that minors could consent to participation in research designed to reduce their personal risk of fatal infection.

Perhaps the thorniest issue we faced was potential observation of criminal activity. We operated under the precept that private citizens have no duty to report criminal activity as long as they neither assist nor encourage it. In contrast, as for child abuse reporting, we counseled interviewers to adhere to Colorado's legal requirements; fortunately, no instance of child abuse was observed during the study interval. Lastly, procedures were implemented to prevent inadvertent disclosure of information such as might occur in a car accident (interview records transported by field investigators) or in the office (access by unauthorized personnel, cleaning crew, burglars).

4.5.4 Data management and security

The collection of sensitive behavioral data from, and description of links between, persons from stigmatized populations placed data security as a high priority concern. Few people had access to our data. Project staff were full-time, trusted employees of the health department. To reduce risk of disclosure the respondent data sheet, which contained identifying information on participants, had potentially incriminating information about respondents recorded below a dotted line. The unique study number assigned to questionnaires was stamped at both top and bottom of the respondent data sheet. This meant that identifying information could be removed by cutting each sheet in two along the dotted line, permitting the sensitive portion of the records to be stored in a secure location. Similarly, the behavioral section of the questionnaire was designed for separation of responses from respondent identity. Name listings contained occupation; to eliminate recording potentially incriminating data, interviewers were instructed to substitute euphemisms for illicit occupations. For example, drug dealers were coded as "sales" persons; genuine salespeople were coded in a manner that made their occupations clear in the analyses.

After participants were assigned unique network identifiers, untraceable to personally identifying information, the data security protocol called for permanent destruction of personal data from hard copy and electronic records, including signed consent forms, thus preventing possible misuse.

4.5.4.1 Database architecture

The initial electronic database consisted of a simple spreadsheet listing study subjects and their partners. In mid-1989, an attempt was made to depict connected persons on a large sheet of paper. It was this manual exercise that provided the ideas for the design of a user-friendly set of databases; these were organized with two goals in mind: separating personal identifiers from potentially compromising information (e.g. sexual practices or illegal behavior), and maintaining the identities of respondents separate from those of the partners they named. Data were entered, using Advanced DB Master software on a 386 IBM-compatible computer, in six flat-file databases. They were designed during the first half of 1989 and contained, respectively: (*a*) respondent identifiers, (*b*) partner identifiers, (*c*) blood test results, (*d*) self-reported knowledge and behaviors, (*e*) relational information between respondents and their partners, and (f) relational information between the partners themselves. Although we perceived no realistic threat to our data's security, we felt it prudent to create a code (termed X-XY-Y, or "XY" for short) to provide a random correspondence between two sets of numbers and to generate unique primary identifiers in the databases. For example, person A was identified by the number X in one table and his or her activities (e.g. drug use) by Y in another table. Possession of the XY code key was necessary to link specific persons with their specific activities: one half of the XY code was linked to respondents; the other half to named partners and the respondents' behavioral information. Electronic copies of the XY code were scrambled with DES encryption, and only two copies of the code were retained on paper. In case of threats to security, paper copies of the XY code could be cut in two; the portion containing personal identifiers could thus be shipped to a safe location. Disk utilities were used to erase copies linking-identifying information from computer hard drives. Data were reviewed for completeness and accuracy and entered in the appropriate databases by the data entry clerk, using the paper copy of the XY code to obtain the primary identifiers for entry. Respondent data sheets, consent forms, and survey instruments were stored in physically separate locations.

In due course our database software became powerful enough to accommodate relational files. This substantially reduced data entry time and minimized errors caused by use of a paper copy of the XY code; this code itself was incorporated into a database and placed onto a floppy disk. The relational databases were structured in such a way that the XY code floppy disk was the key permitting the relational database system to function (Klovdahl 1995).

One of the first removable hard drives manufactured for personal computers was used in this project. Whenever leaving the office, the hard drive would be removed from the computer and hidden in a locked file cabinet within a locked closet. The diskette containing the XY code key was stored separately from both the removable hard drives and the system backup discs. Importantly, the project data analysis computer was not a part of any network. Internet access was provided through a Unix shell on the mainframe of a local university; access was achieved by dialing out over phone lines. When not in use, the phone line was disconnected from the computer's modem, guarding against the event of modem failure (accepting an incoming call). Computer repairs were done in-house, failed hard drives burned, and failing XY floppy disks destroyed. These procedures enhanced data security, yet we recognized that none could be entirely fail-safe.

4.5.4.2 Name matching and de-duplication
The study's recruitment design required that cross-links, persons named by two or more study subjects, be screened for eligibility for the study and subsequent enrollment. Thus, the first goal of our computerized data storage and analysis capability was timely and accurate identification of named partners who were themselves respondents, and of partners who were linked to two or more respondents. To minimize partner duplication, we compiled corroborative sociodemographic

identifying information on each individual, whether respondent or partner. Criteria for matching information included name and alias, residence, site of association, telephone number, occupation, physical characteristics, vehicle ownership, and so on. Telephone directories, including reverse directories, and our STD/HIV Program databases were used to verify or supplement identifying information. SAS (SAS 1985) was used to merge pertinent information from the databases and to sort and print it.

Until recently, name-matching was conducted manually, consuming weeks of tedious labor. At the time (late 1980s, early 1990s) we knew of no inexpensive, DOS PC-based software that could perform this critical function; fuzzy matching techniques were in their infancy. De-duplicating individual namings was complicated by the frequently anonymous nature of contact between prostitutes and their clients, and by their being reported by street name, nickname, or alias. Consequently, databases were designed to contain up to nine first and nine last names. SAS list-generation routines first appended respondent and partner descriptors to one data set, then permutated each observation by all combinations of first and last name before sorting. Overall, four different types of outputs were created: a last name, a first name, a phone number, and an address, sort. Name sorts included sorts by various spellings. Highlighters were used to indicate possible matches on printed lists. Candidates for de-duplication were reviewed by more than one person to assess likely matches. A second unique identifier (network node number) was created to keep track of persons classified as unique individuals. Node number sorts were generated to minimize risk of misnumbering individuals. Lastly, unique sequential node numbers were divided into two separate ranges: the numbers 1 through 9999 were reserved for positively identified persons, and numbers greater than 9999, for those who were not. After the end of each list-generation cycle, printed name lists were shredded and computer files containing merged information from the databases were wiped from the hard drives.

4.6 METHODOLOGICAL ISSUES

4.6.1 Network analysis and visualization in the early years

As of 1989, the main network analysis program for personal computers was UCINET (Borgatti et al. 1999); unfortunately it was not yet capable of accommodating network data exceeding 150 nodes. Accordingly, data sets comprising individuals identified only by number were sent via the Internet to Klovdahl, who worked in Australia. There, his MacroNet program (Klovdahl and Omodei 1978), which could be dimensioned to handle very large networks, was used to examine network connectedness and to generate indices of centrality. The first computer runs of our data were completed in mid-1989; preliminary results were reported shortly thereafter (Woodhouse et al. 1990, 1991). This initial (Year 1 interviews) network comprised 142 respondents and their named partners (557 individuals—network nodes—in all, including one HIV-positive person), with 81 (57 percent) of respondents forming one large connected component. Visualizing this large network in three dimensions was made possible using programs written by Klovdahl, who was inspired by computer programs used to visualize chemical molecules, especially large proteins (Klovdahl 1981, 1986). Node identifiers, along with selected network indices, were processed on a supercomputer at the Australian National University, where multi-dimensional scaling (MDS) routines were used to convert connection information and graph-theoretic distances into coordinates in three-dimensional space. These MDS coordinates pulled network nodes that were near to each other, via shortest paths, closer together in the visual representations; thus crossings of lines were minimized. The result could be viewed locally using the United States Air Force Academy's Evans & Sutherland graphics workstation and Klovdahl's View_Net program (Klovdahl 1986), which could rotate, scale, and edit network visuals in real time. (Thanks to our neighbors at the US Air Force Academy, we were able to view, in late 1990 and early 1991, our evolving networks in three dimensions on hardware used for flight-training.) Hard copies of network visual representations were plotted using a chemical molecule plotting program (ORTEP) (Klovdahl 1981). One such representation is presented in Fig. 4.1.

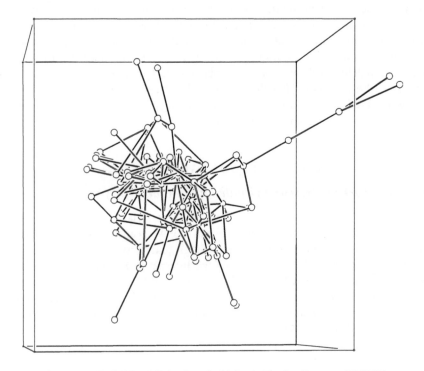

Figure 4.1. *Early Visual Using Protein Molecule Plotting Program (ORTEP)*

4.6.2 Network analysis in the later years

As the magnitude of the data set increased, transferring depersonalized information via the Internet with the available (2400 baud) modem became cumbersome. Our continuing search for more powerful software for desktop computers led us, in mid-1991, to a remarkable program: GRADAP (GRaph Analysis and Definition Package) (Inter-University Project Group of the Universities of Amsterdam 1989). It was capable of performing specific network analyses on large data sets through clever use of hard drive resources. Though GRADAP was constrained by the 640k DOS memory barrier, it was capable of performing distance-based calculations on networks with as many as 6000 nodes and 60,000 connections. GRADAP describes a social network in graph theoretic terms as a set of points and lines, delineates existing connections between individuals, and groups individuals into discrete components (persons connected to each other by at least one path of some length). It is designed to generate key mathematical indices of network structure.

By 1991, our data set contained information on nearly 7000 persons (nodes) comprising respondents, partners, and associates. The principal analytic difficulty was trying to make sense of the results; consequently, ways to make complexity manageable were sought. It seemed that network regions of greatest interest could be conceptualized as cage-like structures—portions of networks that formed closed cycles. While it seemed to us that branching sections of the networks were less likely to promote sustained transmission of pathogens (because branches eventually led to termini), it also seemed likely that looping regions could form efficient transmission pathways. A graph theory technique, stepwise reduction, was used to remove terminal branches in stepwise fashion until only closed loops remained (Centers for Disease Control and Prevention 1993; Potterat et al. 1996). Unfortunately, when attempting to use GRADAP to reduce our networks, its limitations were reached. Due to the limited importance attached by funding bodies to computer program development for social sciences research, our European colleagues were not able to obtain the support necessary to revise and extend their innovative program. From that point, we were compelled to create complex SAS routines to progress.

4.6.3 Obstacles and solutions

The Colorado Springs staff seriously underestimated the complexity of analyzing social network data and overestimated the stamina of sponsoring agencies and potential consultants. Quite aside from the fact that network analysis programs for personal computers were either unavailable or not powerful enough to accommodate large data sets in the early years, the project's future was jeopardized by CDC's waning interest in the wake of Darrow's departure as project officer. In mid-1991, the CDC began to press the Colorado Springs staff to bring the project to an end and to generate manuscripts for submission to professional journals; unfortunately, neither staff nor analytic results were ready for these ambitions at this point. Network analyses are more intensive than analyses of characteristics of individuals. Operationally, the staff was directed to terminate enrollment of baseline respondents and to concentrate on increasing the number of interviews on follow-up, cross-link, and HIV-positive, participants.

Specialized consultants who in the early years had promised to assist with the advanced analyses were, by the time data collection was 3 years old, committed elsewhere. It was at this point that a long-term colleague, Richard Rothenberg, provided assistance with advanced analyses. At the same time that CDC was losing interest in the Colorado Springs project, the National Institute on Drug Abuse (NIDA) was being introduced to the social network paradigm. A NIDA technical review session was held in 1991 "to stimulate researchers to use network analysis . . . to explore HIV-related behavioral transactions" (Trotter et al. 1995). By the mid-1990s, NIDA expressed interest in our data sets and encouraged us to apply for funding; the Colorado Springs project received a $366,456 2-year grant to procure technical assistance.

Clearly, anyone contemplating the collection of social network data should be aware of the complexity, time, and costs involved. It is also important to insure that all information contained in these complex data is examined; they promise new insights into problems of importance to society (e.g. infectious disease propagation). Indeed, not to take advantage of data collected is to seriously undervalue the cooperation of study participants, who are at the very least owed the courtesy of fully exploring their contribution. In addition, being able to tap into a range of expert help is necessary to avoid pitfalls suggested by Woody Allen's aphorism: "Autodidacts have the worst teachers."

4.7 ILLUSTRATIVE FINDINGS

Because development of survey instruments and pilot testing consumed nearly 6 months, recruitment of participants did not begin until May 1988. Recruitment of new participants ended in August 1991 (Muth et al. 1992). Of the 1079 eligible persons identified during this interval, 595 (55 percent) were enrolled. Of eligible persons not enrolled, most (384/484) could not be located—a consequence of the frequently peripatetic nature of the populations of interest—or were not approached for confidentiality reasons, while 28 percent (136/484) refused to participate. In 1091 interviews overall, respondents named 8164 network associates in a community of nearly 400,000 persons. (In total, over the duration of the entire study, 8759 unique individuals were found to be connected by 31,147 links.) These 1091 interviews included 595 baseline interviews, and 288 second, 135 third, and 73 fourth/fifth, wave interviews.

As detailed in the first column of Table 4.1, the proportion of participants in each of the major recruitment categories changed during the 4 years of baseline enrollment.

The proportion of prostitute women declined during the last 2 years, while the proportion of IDU increased during the same period. Attrition of follow-up interviews was associated with respondent mobility and project resource limitations, rather than with respondent refusal to continue with the study. During the study interval, attrition tended to be stable among prostitute women and high among their

Table 4.1. *Recruitment and Attrition in Four Cohorts of Study Respondents in Colorado Springs, 1988–92*

Recruitment period	Recruitment category	Wave											Total	
		1		2		3		4		5				
		N	%	N	%	N	%	N	%	N	%	N	%
Year 1	Prostitute	47	44	35	55	28	60	23	66	1	25	134	52
	Partner	38	35	15	23	7	15	4	11	1	25	65	25
	IDU	20	19	14	22	12	26	8	23	2	50	56	22
	Other	3	3	0	0	0	0	0	0	0	0	3	1
	Total	108	100	64	100	47	100	35	100	4	100	258	100
Year 2	Prostitute	32	23	23	24	17	28	10	29			82	25
	Partner	51	36	32	34	18	30	9	26			110	33
	IDU	40	28	25	27	15	25	9	26			89	27
	Other	19	13	14	15	10	17	6	18			49	15
	Total	142	100	94	100	60	100	34	100			330	100
Year 3	Prostitute	42	17	21	17	9	32					72	18
	Partner	68	28	32	26	7	25					107	27
	IDU	99	40	53	44	9	32					161	41
	Other	38	15	15	12	3	11					56	14
	Total	247	100	121	100	28	100					396	100
Year 4	Prostitute	12	12	0	0							12	11
	Partner	20	20	2	22							22	21
	IDU	40	41	5	26							45	42
	Other	26	27	2	22							28	26
	Total	98	100	9	100							107	100
Total	Prostitute	133	22	79	27	54	40	33	48	1	25	300	27
	Partner	177	30	81	28	32	24	13	19	1	25	304	28
	IDU	199	33	97	34	36	27	17	25	2	50	351	32
	Other*	86	14	31	11	13	10	6	9	0	0	136	12
	Total	595	100	288	100	135	100	69	100	4	100	1091	100

* Other (*N* = 86) comprises thirty-nine cross-link- (see text), forty-one sex partner of IDU-, and six miscellaneous-respondents.

partners, and tended to be high among IDU during the latter years (Table 4.1, row data, and Table 4.2).

Network analysis revealed that most individuals (7151 of 8759, or 82 percent) comprised a single connected component, with each being connected to every other person by at least one path of some length; in addition, there were 116 smaller components with no observed links to the largest component. Of the 31,147 total links, roughly one-fifth of known relationships (5502/29,835) between respondents and their partners could be classified as risky for HIV transmission (Table 4.3).

As reported elsewhere, risk network analysis showed that seventeen (3 percent) respondents were HIV-positive, of whom only one was assessed to have acquired HIV during the observation period. The single largest risk component contained eight HIV-positives, with the other nine located in small components (Darrow et al. 1999). Although partners of respondents were not sought for HIV testing, availability of our HIV/AIDS surveillance database provided the opportunity to match names of partners against those with known HIV infection. As of the end of 1999, seventeen partners named by respondents were also known to be HIV-infected, as were two study-eligible persons (neither interviewed nor named by other respondents), for a total of thirty-six HIV-infected persons in our cohort. Twenty-five of these thirty-six

Table 4.2. *Percentage of Respondents Recaptured for Subsequent Interviews, by Wave, Colorado Springs, 1988–92*

Recruitment period	Recruitment category	Wave		
		2	3	4
Year 1	Prostitute	74	60	49
	Partner	39	18	11
	IDU	70	60	40
	Other	0	0	0
	Total	59	44	32
Year 2	Prostitute	72	53	31
	Partner	63	35	18
	IDU	63	38	23
	Other	74	53	32
	Total	66	42	24
Year 3	Prostitute	50	21	
	Partner	47	10	
	IDU	53	9	
	Other	39	8	
	Total	49	11	
Year 4	Prostitute	0		
	Partner	10		
	IDU	13		
	Other	8		
	Total	9		

Note: IDU, injecting drug use.

Table 4.3. *Hierarchical[a] Distribution of Network Links, by Category in Colorado Springs, 1988–92*

Risk gradient[a]	Links	
	N	%
IDU	1246	4
Sexual	4256	14
Drug use	9245	31
Social	15,088	51
Unknown[b]	1312	NA
Total	31,147	100

[a] Multiple links were counted only once using the risk gradient (from highest to lowest) in column one.
[b] Excluded from the denominator.

persons are embedded in a network comprised of recent risky contacts: 3210 persons for whom vaginal/anal sex or/and needle-sharing contact occurred within 6 months of interview (Fig. 4.2). The largest black circles indicate HIV-infected persons, medium-size white circles indicate persons without HIV infection, and the smallest dots indicate persons for whom HIV serostatus is unknown. Interconnecting lines represent vaginal, anal or/and needle-sharing contact between persons. A large connected component of 2004 persons (16 with HIV, 328 without, 1660 unknown) is apparent at the top of the figure, while the remaining 1206 persons (9 with HIV, 247 without, 950 unknown) are scattered towards the bottom in 223 small components, ranging in size from two to twenty-four persons.

Notably, while HIV-infected persons had a non-significant tendency to reside in the large (4.7 percent) versus the small (3.5 percent) components (odds ratio = 1.34; 95 percent confidence interval 0.55–3.34; $P = 0.49$), those within the large component were shown to occupy peripheral positions. Although this discovery was initially made using numerical measures of centrality, direct visual confirmation can be realized through the technique of stepwise graph reduction.

Figure 4.3 illustrates three stages in the graph reduction process: (*a*) the first round of reduction where singly connected nodes are removed, (*b*) the fifth round of reduction, where remaining persons connect to at least two others (a "2-core"), and (*c*) the 18th round of reduction, where remaining persons connect to at least three others (a "3-core"). Of the sixteen HIV-infected persons in the largest component, eleven remain after a single round of reduction (Fig. 3(a)), and only two remain after five rounds (Fig. 3(b)). No HIV-infected persons are evident among sixty-nine persons in the stepwise-reduced 3-core (Fig. 3(c)), the heart of the risk network. For reasons not entirely clear, HIV infection in Colorado Springs never reached the central core of the network and hence could not be expected to propagate into the rest of the network and into the larger community. This observation probably best explains the dearth of HIV incidence observed during the study interval (Potterat et al. 1993).

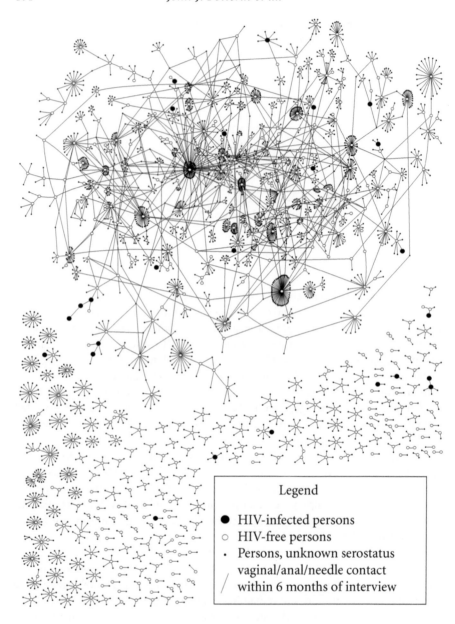

Figure 4.2. *Network Location of HIV-infected Persons*

The 133 enrolled prostitute women represent three-fifths of the 217 we identified during the enrollment period, while the 766 IDUs identified as a consequence of network namings represent about half of the estimated 1500 current injectors, a crude estimate projected from national estimates published in the early 1990s.

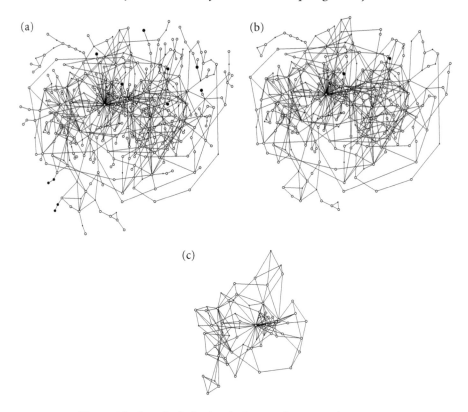

Figure 4.3. *Stepwise Reduction, by Degree of Largest Risk-component*

The project's prospective design provided the opportunity to study the changing character of networks over time. We knew that our purposive sampling design might affect generalizability and complicate assessment of the reliability of observed changes. To assess the changing size and shape of networks over time while minimizing bias, we used data from the two cohorts of respondents for whom we had three cumulative years of regularly spaced interviews (Rothenberg et al. 1998). Changes in partnership formation, in risk behavior configuration, and in network structure were examined. Although differences were noted in each cohort, overall results suggested diminution of risk on the part of respondents who remained with the project during the 3-year interval. The stability of networks varied with the type of relationship; stability was defined as the proportion of all individuals nominated at two successive time points who were nominated at both time points. In general, for both cohorts, sexual and social networks became more stable (i.e. low actor turn-over) over time, drug-using partnerships remained constant in their low stability, and needle-sharing partnerships remained unstable in one cohort but became somewhat more stable in the second cohort (Rothenberg et al. 1998). Both risk behavior and risk configuration (its social context) changed in the direction of decreasing risk from the first to the third interval, although small differences were noted between the two cohorts. Overall network cohesion decreased over time: the number of separate components increased for risky relationships. In addition, the size of the larger components decreased significantly for all relationships in both cohorts, especially for sex and needle-sharing relationships in the second cohort. These changes both suggest diminution of group interaction (smaller and fewer components). Examination of microstructural elements (cycles) corroborated observations made at the macrostructural (components) level. With few exceptions, all measures of subgroup formation revealed diminution of structural cohesion over time. As we conclude elsewhere,

"the observed changes may have resulted from [our] intervention efforts, or possibly from client contact associated with the study itself. Both are difficult to rule out, and it is possible that program or study factors may have influenced the personal behaviors to which they would have been targeted. The differences in the risk-taking of the two cohorts, in the presence of a constant program effect (no special campaigns) speaks against such impact. In addition, it is unlikely that program intervention would have had direct effect on the observed changes in network structure. The fact that such change may take place spontaneously in a group at presumptive risk is a cautionary note for evaluation of an intervention's impact." (Rothenberg et al. 1998)

Location and prominence of HIV-positive persons within networks was examined using eight measures of centrality (Rothenberg et al. 1995), because we viewed such network properties as a surrogate for disease transmission potential. Although these centrality measures differ theoretically and computationally, their application to our data produced similar results. We used GRADAP to assess measures related to distance, adjacency, and betweenness. Distance measures how close a person is to others in the network; adjacency, the opportunity for direct connection to others; and betweenness, the opportunity for a person to act as a barrier or a conduit. Assuming that these measures are directly related to probability of disease transmission, they confirmed the non-centrality of HIV-positive persons in our network, thus helping to account for the lack of observed HIV transmission.

4.7.1 Lessons learned

The crucial initial finding was that members of stigmatized groups in Colorado Springs—many of whose behaviors were illegal—were willing to provide complete identifying information on their social, drug, and sexual partners for research purposes. Expecting members of marginalized populations to provide such information for disease control purposes may have been rational, based on previous experience, yet willingness to cooperate in the absence of disease was unexpected. We believe that their cooperation was due to the trust our staff earned through sustained and sympathetic outreach efforts prior to and during the study. Thus, we learned that contact interviewing could succeed even in the absence of sexually transmissible or blood-borne infection; properly approached, members of our study populations willingly revealed the most intimate secrets of their lives. Moreover, we have no evidence that confidential HIV testing or solicitation of full identifiers on partners deterred enroll-ment of respondents, or discouraged their full participation.

For us, the most critical issue is how completely the observed social network picture corresponds to reality. We found that most respondents and their named partners could ultimately be connected into a single large component. To what extent, however, is the existence of many smaller components an artifact of lacunae in data collection? The fact that no demonstrable link to the largest component was observed for about 30 percent of respondents and their linked partners could be an artifact of incomplete information. Ideally, we would like to have been able to: (*a*) enroll all eligible respondents, (*b*) recapture nearly all for follow-up interview, (*c*) use an interview period of 1 year instead of 6 months, (*d*) interview all named partners, and (*e*) get respondents with the inclination and ability to list all relevant partners. The question therefore arises: with optimal conditions, would we have observed a similar pattern? Theoretical consideration supports an affirmative answer. In general, persons choose partners very much like themselves (Potterat et al. 1985). It is this pronounced tendency to partner homophily that can be expected to produce discretely bounded subpopulations, at least some of which will not have members forming bridges to subpopulations different from their own. This observa-tion may especially be true of subpopulations some of whose members may suffer from mental illness (Centers for Disease Control and Prevention 1997), such as illicit drug users (Michels and Marzuk 1998), and prostitute women (Potterat et al. 1998). In any event, we speculate that the difference between what we observed and perfect ascertainment is quantitative, not qualitative. Although the fabric is torn and frayed, the underlying picture probably reflects reality.

We used multiple methods for identifying potential respondents, including can-vassing persons appearing in high-risk medical settings for eligibility; conducting continuous street outreach; monitoring lists of partners who were reported by respondents to have engaged in the behaviors of interest; and attempting to enroll persons who were named by at least two separate respondents. This approach is typically used to reach rare or elusive populations (Johnson et al. 1990); it is a mix of systematic sampling, chain-link ascertainment, and purposive sampling. Although nonrandom, resulting samples may yet be assessed as representative by comparing the characteristics of participants with ethnographic observations (Trotter et al. 1995; Rothenberg and Narramore 1996). The overall impression we derive from our project data is that enrolled participants are reasonably representative of the under-lying populations and networks we sought to study (Muth et al. 2000).

The Colorado Springs project was the first prospective study to provide empirical support for the hypothesis that network structure may shape the transmission of sexually transmissible or bloodborne agents. In a recent paper, we concluded that "just as language can be conceptualized as a flow of words structured by rules of grammar, so may epidemics be viewed as a flow of microbes structured by the 'grammar' of social network structures" (Potterat et al. 1999*b*). Although this con-clusion must be viewed with appropriate circumspection because of uncertainties about sampling, error estimation, and data collection limitations, our results and those of others (Trotter et al. 1995; Friedman et al. 1997; Rothenberg et al. 1998) suggest that the study of the influence of network properties in the diffusion of infectious agents is a promising approach for future inquiry—which should include reassessment of the adequacy of the standard STD/HIV reproductive number formula ($R = \beta cD$) to gauge transmission dynamics (Potterat et al. 2000).

Notable was the project's attempt to capture changes in network configuration over time. Observed network dynamism in Colorado Springs provides clearer insight into the possible influence of macro- and micro-structural elements in disease propagation. An area of low HIV prevalence at the start of the study, the dearth of subsequent HIV transmission in Colorado Springs's heterosexual populations may at least in part be related to the lack of network structural features that foster active propagation, despite the continued presence of risky behaviors. The relative contribution of local HIV prevalence, anemic network structure, and risky behavior configuration to observed disease transmission cannot be clearly separated from the available data. Nevertheless, the Colorado Springs data suggest an important role for network architecture in HIV transmission dynamics. Although our observations may be confounded by changes in our sample population over time and by respondent attrition, it is of interest that configuration of macro- and micro-structural network properties were also strongly associated with observed syphilis transmission in a sexual network of heterosexual adolescents in Atlanta during 1996 (Rothenberg et al. 1998). Our overall conclusion is that although risky behaviors are necessary for the transmission of HIV or syphilis, individual behaviors—and indeed, personal networks—alone are not sufficient to explain STD/HIV propagation.

Availability of our relatively large data set afforded the opportunity to empirically test many of the available measures of network prominence. The demonstration that different centrality measures are both robust and comparable was an encouraging finding (Rothenberg et al. 1994). In addition, the preliminary conclusions reached by this study (Woodhouse et al. 1990; Woodhouse et al. 1991; Muth et al. 1992) stimulated, in the early 1990s, the development of newer mathematical models that attempt to factor in network structure (Klovdahl et al. 1992; Potterat et al. 2000).

An important lesson is that we woefully underestimated the amount of interviewer resources necessary to do the job right. The availability of additional resources (e.g. a few more interviewers) would clearly have increased baseline enrollment, the proportion of follow-up interviews, and enrollment of cross-links. Although it is true that eligible respondents move often, movement in Colorado Springs usually occurred within the same few neighborhoods. Our impression is that adequate staffing would have substantially improved enrollment outcomes. Such efforts are especially important in light of our observation that "shortcomings in our data have less to do with reluctance to provide information than with the frequently anonymous nature of sexual encounters" (Rothenberg et al. 1994). The wider one can cast the net, the more probable the capture of partners that may have been difficult to be identified due to the anonymous nature of some encounters (Potterat et al. 1989).

Enrolling more respondents would have improved risk behavior validity assessment. As it is, risk behaviors were unilaterally reported by respondents, and there were few opportunities other than by ethnography to corroborate these self-reports. In addition, use of the relatively short (6-months) interview period, combined with the fact that we did not request dates of exposure (only that exposure occurred within that interval), renders assessment of directionality impossible. Directionality is theoretically important to map the potential flow of STD/HIV microbes via sexual or parenteral routes (e.g. are partners upstream or downstream?).

The Colorado Springs project failed to consider the impact on potential transmission occasioned by periods of confinement, due either to incarceration or drug rehabilitation. No question in any part of the survey instrument requested this information. Members of both prostitute and injecting drug-using populations commonly face confinement where, presumably, opportunities for continuance of risky behaviors are constrained, if not eliminated. Controlling for such potential gaps in exposure would seem to be important in the analysis of constraints to observed transmission that could be misattributed to network configuration. In addition, controlling for extended periods of absence from the Colorado Springs area due to reasons other than forced confinement may have been relevant.

With hindsight, several additional questions may have been useful: to capture data about indirect sharing of drug injection equipment (Koester and Hoffer 1994); to delineate drug of choice in populations of polydrug users; and to describe musical (e.g. Rock 'n Roll, Rap, Country and Western, Jazz, Bluegrass, Folk, Classical, etc.) or (today) web-browsing preferences. Lastly, obtaining better locating information (e.g. "Who else would know where you might be a year from now?") or perhaps attempting a "contractual" arrangement with participants (e.g. "We'll pay you $25 if you call us about 1 year from now, even if you choose not to participate") may have improved respondent recapture rates.

We were fortunate to retain trained and motivated project staff for long periods; employee stability was a hallmark of the Colorado Springs STD/HIV program during the last three decades of the twentieth century. It is our opinion that many of the obstacles we encountered were minimized because of staff attributes: persistence, dedication, and enthusiasm. Researchers contemplating the challenging tasks of collecting, collating, and analyzing network data longitudinally must consider the probably deleterious effect of staff turnover, as well as possible burnout or disenchantment.

4.7.2 Work in progress

Of paramount interest to both researchers and field workers are economical ways to rapidly and reliably assess network structure. Development of user-friendly network sampling techniques would also serve to encourage investigators who are interested in network studies but who are discouraged by the daunting task of full-network ascertainment. Efforts are currently underway to analyze our data to determine the minimum required sample necessary to accurately describe network structure. Of particular interest is order of enrollment: are persons who are reached first for participation more likely to occupy a more central role in potential disease transmission than those contacted later in the study?

Of importance as well are explorations of the dynamics of partner selection and mixing patterns. What are the social and geographic determinants of partner selection for sexual or illicit drug use purposes? What are the characteristics of persons bridging disparate groups? For example, what is the geographic distance between persons engaging in different kinds of risky relationships (Fig. 4.4)? Perhaps more importantly, is geographic distance an influential network attribute? Databased answers to such questions will improve our understanding of network boundaries in Colorado Springs's high risk populations.

Comparability of study participants with nonparticipants is usually assessed by contrasting the distributions of sociodemographic characteristics. Such comparisons do not necessarily provide insight into whether or not participants of a given subgroup are similar to nonparticipants of the same subgroup. Geographic data may provide such insight by visually displaying the spatial distributions of participants and nonparticipants. We are exploring spatial analytical methods to assess sampling problems commonly encountered in social network studies, especially techniques that can shed light on sample representativeness (Muth et al. 2000).

A crucial need is development of user-friendly social network analysis software that can accommodate large, real-world networks and produce summary indices of network structure and dynamics with minimal user computer sophistication. To that end, for example, we have recently developed a simpler method for computing some indices of actor prominence, the prestige scores of Katz and Hoede (Foster and Muth et al. 2001), and implemented a technique to delineate components without resorting to computationally intensive matrix-based methods. Importantly, a powerful freeware package for analysis and visualization of very large networks, Pajek, became available on the World Wide Web (http://vlado.fmf.uni-lj.si/pub/networks/pajek) in 1997. Although in the process of continuing development, Pajek's strengths are its advanced network visualization capabilities and its optimized network partitioning algorithms.

4.8 SUMMARY

The Colorado Springs project was a pathbreaking investigation of the influence of network structure on the transmission of sexually or parenterally transmissible agents. Its most remarkable feature is that it was brought to fruition largely by health workers actively involved in disease prevention at the street level, with no formal experience in network analysis. Neither absence of in-house expertise nor inadequacy of personnel resources prevented it from achieving its aims. In retrospect, ignorance of potential obstacles was bliss, for it is unlikely that this project would have been undertaken had the Colorado Springs staff been cognizant of the complexities detailed here. Importantly, at the time, the health department in Colorado Springs was small, independent, and neither hierarchically nor bureaucratically rigid, affording the staff much freedom to experiment with new ideas and approaches. Moreover, the idea of entrusting the task of delineating network structure in heterosexual

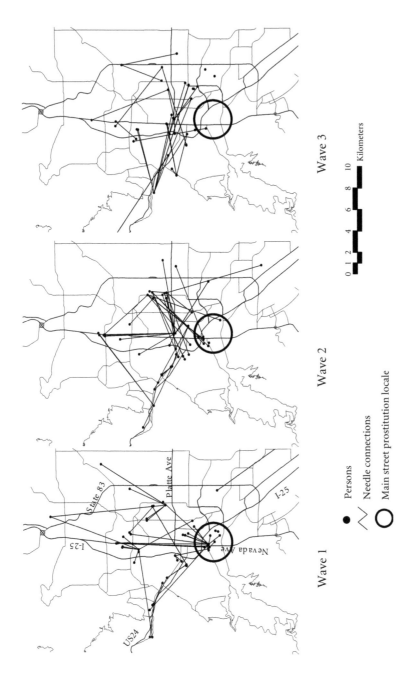

Wave 1   Wave 2   Wave 3

•   Persons

⋀   Needle connections

◯   Main street prostitution locale

0 1 2   4   6   8   10   Kilometers

Figure 4.4. *Needle-sharing Connections in Geographic (Residential) Space*

populations at risk for HIV to STD contact tracers was probably appropriate, for such health workers have long understood the importance of social context in disease transmission and frequently have the trust of the populations of interest.

Although our data strongly support Klovdahl's premise that network structure affects infectious disease transmission, health department workers may be tempted to claim credit for the observed lack of HIV transmission in Colorado Springs during the study interval (Woodhouse et al. 1994; Rothenberg et al. 1996). After all, the project included built-in intervention efforts with study participants in context of ongoing community-wide STD/HIV interventions. We remind ourselves that caution suggests assessing the impact of program interventions as modest. Spontaneous changes in network structure may occur frequently in populations such as the ones we studied. The truly important conclusion is that network configuration was, as predicted by theory, associated with observed patterns of disease propagation, irrespective of what may have caused those changes—public health interventions or inherent structural dynamism or both. Though the network approach to infectious disease epidemiology may indeed be revolutionary, considerably more research is needed to understand the forces that underlie network dynamics before we can more confidently design public health interventions aimed at inhibiting the spread of infectious disease.

References

Auerbach, D., Darrow, W. et al. (1984). "Cluster of cases of the acquired immune deficiency syndrome. Patients linked by sexual contact," *Am J Med*, 76(3): 487–92.

Borgatti, S., Everett, M. et al. (1999). *UCINET 5.0 Version 1.00 for Windows: Software for Social Network Analysis*. Harvard, MA: Natick Analytic Technologies.

Centers for Disease Control and Prevention (1987). "Antibody to human immunodeficiency virus in female prostitutes," *Morbid Mortal Weekly Rep*, 36: 157–61.

—— (1992). "Street outreach for STD/HIV prevention—Colorado Springs, Colorado," *Morbid Mortal Weekly Rep*, 41(6): 94–5, 101.

—— (1993). "Gang-related outbreak of penicillinase-producing Neisseria gonorrhoeae and other sexually transmitted diseases—Colorado Springs, 1989–1991," *Morbid Mortal Weekly Rep*, 42(2): 25–8.

—— (1997). "Community-based HIV prevention in presumably underserved populations—Colorado Springs, Colorado, July–September 1995," *Morbid Mortal Weekly Rep*, 46: 152–5.

Darrow, W., Potterat, J. et al. (1999). "Using knowledge of social networks to prevent human immunodeficiency virus infections: The Colorado Springs study," *Soc Focus*, 32: 143–58.

Foster, K., Muth, S. et al. (2001). "A faster Katz status score algorithm," *Comput Math Org Theory*, 7: 275–85.

Frank, O. (1978). "Sampling and estimation in large social networks," *Soc Networks*, 1: 91–101.

Friedman, S. R., Neaigus, A. et al. (1997). "Sociometric risk networks and HIV risk," *Am J Public Health*, 87(8): 1289–96.

Inter-University Project Group of the Universities of Amsterdam, Groningen, Nijmegen, and Twente (1989). *GRADAP: Graph Definition and Analysis Package*, Groningen: ProGamma.

Johnson, A. M., Wadsworth, J. et al. (1990). "Surveying sexual attitudes," *Nature*, 343: 109.

Johnson, J. (1990). "Selecting ethnographic informants," A Sage University Paper. *Qualitative Research Methods Series No. 22*. Newbury Park, CA: Sage.

Khabbaz, R., Darrow, W. et al. (1990). "Seroprevalence and risk factors for HTLV-I/II infection among female prostitutes in the United States," *JAMA*, 163: 60–4.

Klovdahl, A. (1981). "A note on images of networks," *Soc Networks*, 3: 197–214.

—— (1986). "View_Net: A new tool for network analysis," *Soc Networks*, 8: 313–42.

—— (1989). "Urban social networks: Some methodological problems and possibilities." In M. Kochen (ed.), *The Small World* (Norwood, NJ), pp. 176–210.

—— (1995). "Levels of protection: Confidentiality in network research," *Bull Meth Soc*, 48: 120–32.

—— Dhofier, Z. et al. (1977). "Social networks in an urban area: First Canberra study." *Austr N Z J Soc*, 13: 169–75.

—— and Omodei, R. (1978). "Macronet: A set of programs for computing symmetric adjacency, reachability and distance matrices for larger networks," *Connections*, 1(2): 19.

—— Potterat, J. et al. (1992). "HIV infection in an urban social network: A progress report," *Bull Meth Soc*, 36: 24–33.

Klovdahl, A. S. (1985). "Social networks and the spread of infectious diseases. The AIDS example," *Soc Sci Med*, 21(11): 1203–16.

—— Potterat, J. J. et al. (1994). "Social networks and infectious disease: The Colorado Springs Study," *Soc Sci Med*, 38(1): 79–88.

Koester, S. and Hoffer, L. (1994). "'Indirect sharing': Additional risks associated with drug injection," *AIDS Pub Pol J*, 9: 100–5.

Michels, R. and Marjun, P. M. (1998). "Progress in psychiatry," *N Engl J Med*, 329: 552–7.

Muth, S., Potterat, J. et al. (2000). "Birds of a feather: Using a rotational box plot to assess ascertainment bias," *Int J Epidemiol*, 29: 899–904.

—— Woodhouse, D. E. et al. (1992). "HIV infection within networks of prostitute women and injecting drug users." Eighth International Conference on AIDS/Third STD World Congress, Amsterdam, July (Abstract THC 1519).

Plummer, L., Potterat, J. et al. (1996). "Providing support and assistance for low-income or homeless women," *JAMA*, 276: 1874–5.

Potterat, J. (1987). "The AIDS epidemic and media coverage: A critical review," *Critique*, 26: 36–8.

—— Muth, J. et al. (1986). "Serological markers as indicators of sexual orientation in AIDS-virus infected men," *JAMA*, 256: 712.

—— Muth, S. et al. (1996). "Chronicle of a gang STD outbreak foretold," *Free Inquir Creative Soc*, 24: 11–16.

—— —— et al. (2000). "Evidence undermining the adequacy of the HIV reproductive number formula," *Sex Transm Dis*, 27: 644–5.

—— Phillips, L. et al. (1985). "On becoming a prostitute: An exploratory case-comparison study," *J Sex Res*, 21: 329–35.

—— —— et al. (1987). "Lying to military physicians about risk factors for HIV infections," *JAMA*, 257: 1727.

—— Rothenberg, R. et al. (1979). "Gonorrhea in street prostitutes: Epidemiologic and legal implications," *Sex Transm Dis*, 6(2): 58–63.

—— —— et al. (1998). "Pathways to prostitution: The chronology of sexual and drug abuse milestones," *J Sex Res*, 35: 333–40.

—— —— (1999a). "Invoking, monitoring and relinquishing a public health power: The Health Hold Order," *Sex Transm Dis*, 26: 345–9.

Potterat, J., Rothenberg, R. et al. (1999*b*). "Network structural dynamics and infectious disease propagation," *AIDS*, 10: 182–5.

—— Spencer, N. et al. (1989). "Partner notification in the control of human immunodeficiency virus infection," *Am J Public Health*, 79: 874–6.

Potterat, J. J., Meheus, A. et al. (1991). "Partner notification: Operational considerations," *Int J STD AIDS*, 2: 411–15.

—— Rothenberg, R. B. et al. (1985). "Gonorrhoea as a social disease," *Sex Trans Dis*, 12: 25–32.

—— Woodhouse, D. E. et al. (1990). "Estimating the prevalence and career longevity of prostitute women." *J Sex Res*, 27(2): 233–43.

—— —— et al. (1993). "AIDS in Colorado Springs: Is there an epidemic?" *AIDS* 7(11): 1517–21.

Rothenberg, R. and Narramore, J. (1996). "The relevance of social network concepts to sexually transmitted disease control," *Sex Transm Dis*, 23(1): 24–9.

—— Potterat, J. et al. (1994). *Choosing a Centrality Measure: Epidemiologic Correlates in the Colorado Springs Study of Social Networks*. New Orleans, LA: Sunbelt Social Network Conference.

—— —— et al. (1995). "Choosing a centrality measure: Epidemiologic correlates in the Colorado Springs study of social networks," *Soc Net*, 17: 273–97.

—— —— et al. (1996). "Personal risk taking and the spread of disease: Beyond core groups," *J Infect Dis* 174(Supp. 2): S144–9.

—— Sterk, C. et al. (1998). "Using social network and ethnographic tools to evaluate syphilis transmission," *Sex Transm Dis*, 25(3): 154–60.

Rothenberg, R. B. (1983). "The geography of gonorrhea: Empirical demonstration of core group transmission," *Am J Epidemiol*, 117: 688–94.

—— Potterat, J. J. et al. (1998). "Social network dynamics and HIV transmission," *AIDS*, 12(12): 1529–36.

SAS, I. I. (1985). *SAS User's Guide: Statistics, Version 5 Edition*. Cary, SAS Institute Inc.

Trotter, R., Bowen, A. et al. (1995). "Network models for HIV outreach and prevention programs for drug users." In R. Needle, S. Coyle, S. Genser, and I. R. Trotter (eds.), *Social Networks, Drug Abuse and HIV Transmission. NIDA Research Monograph 151* (Rockville, MD: National Institute on Drug Abuse), pp. 144–80.

—— Rothenberg, R. et al. (1995). "Drug abuse and HIV prevention research: Expanding paradigms and network contributions to risk reduction," *Connections*, 18: 29–45.

Woodhouse, D., Potterat, L. et al. (1985). "A civilian-military partnership for the reduction of gonorrhea incidence," *Public Health Rep*, 100: 61–5.

—— —— et al. (1990). "Social networks in the transmission of HIV infection." Sixth International Conference on AIDS, San Francisco (Abstract S.C. 679).

—— —— et al. (1991). "HIV infection within networks of prostitute women and intravenous drug users." Seventh International Conference on AIDS, Florence, June (Abstract W.C. 100).

—— —— et al. (1995). "Ethical and legal issues in social networks research: The real and the ideal." In R. Needle, S. Genser, and I. R. Trotter (eds.), *Social Networks, Drug Abuse and HIV Transmission. National Institute on Drug Abuse Monograph No. 151*. NIH Publication No. 95-3889, pp. 131–43.

Woodhouse, D. E., Rothenberg, R. B. et al. (1994). "Mapping a social network of heterosexuals at high risk for HIV infection," *AIDS* 8(9): 1331–6.

5

The Urban and Rural Networks Project: Atlanta and Flagstaff

RICHARD ROTHENBERG, DAVID LONG, CLAIRE STERK, AL PACH,
ROBERT TROTTER, JULIE BALDWIN, AND CAROL MAXWELL

5.1 INTRODUCTION

The Urban and Rural Networks Project was begun as a joint project in Flagstaff AZ (R. Trotter, PI) and Atlanta, GA (R. Rothenberg, PI) to examine the relationship between network structures and dynamics and potential transmission of Human immunodeficiency virus (HIV). Both projects were funded by National Institute on Drug Abuse, NIH as part of an interactive investigator initiated research project grant (IRPG), a mechanism that permits sharing of resources between two or more projects, but retains independent review of each. The projects intended to follow the same network design, and used virtually identical survey and interview instruments. However, the designs diverged during implementation, and though some of the material obtained was comparable, the projects as a whole were not. This discussion will focus primarily on the Atlanta project, with some material from Flagstaff.

These projects owe their genesis to the earlier work in Colorado Springs involving persons at high risk for HIV in an area with low prevalence and low endemic transmission (J. Potterat, PI). The intent of the Urban and Rural Networks project was to examine network structures in areas of lower (Flagstaff) and higher (Atlanta) HIV prevalence.

5.2 SAMPLE

5.2.1 The Chain-Link design

The underlying design (Fig. 5.1) was a Chain-Link sampling approach. First, the "seeds" for each chain were identified. A seed was defined as a person who met certain eligibility criteria, was stable in the community, and was amenable to participation. The seeds for the six chains in Atlanta were all over 18 years of age and active drug users (either crack or heroin injection). The seeds and all of their contacts were

This report is prepared by Richard Rothenberg, David Long, and Al Pach, with review and contribution from other project members.

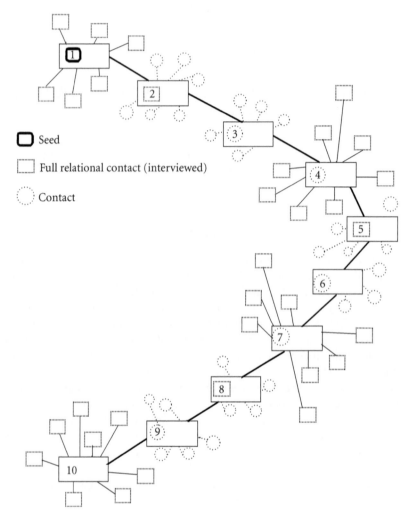

Figure 5.1. *Study Design for Urban and Rural Networks Projects*

interviewed for the study. Enrollment of these contacts for participation in the study was by one of two methods: either the next participant was chosen randomly from among the contacts (Random Walk) or was nominated by the seed (Chain Link). Three of the six community chains were generated by Random Walk and three by Chain Link. For each chain, a total of ten primary, connected responders was chosen. All of the contacts to the first (seed), fourth, seventh, and tenth respondent were also interviewed and their contacts elicited.

The study design was thus a Chain Link approach, as noted, but had the addition of a partial snowball design. The latter portion, limited by available resources, was an attempt to provide a larger sample of the community represented by the initial respondents, and to provide additional data for analysis.

5.2.2 Field sites

The study targeted locations with an identified prevalence of drug distribution and use, particularly "hard" drugs that could be used intravenously (e.g. heroin, methamphetamine, and powder cocaine) or smoked (i.e. crack cocaine). The communities in which the field sites were located maintained a consistently high level of activity throughout the day. This included the normal level of occupational and leisure pursuits, but also included an extensive parallel economy comprising illicit activities such as drug use, drug sales, prostitution, and a variety of other "hustles." As a result, the police maintained a constant presence, and arrests were frequent. In addition, due to the endemic level of poverty many local residents were in constant housing transition and several community services dedicated to the large urban homeless population were located near the field sites. Frequent incarceration of respondents did interfere with follow-up efforts, although research staff were able to conduct interviews in jail on multiple occasions. There were three field sites in the study, although staff would frequently visit peripheral communities connected to the study sites via respondents' social networks. Two field sites were located in the community called the Old Fourth Ward, and a third site was located in the Mechanicsville community.

5.2.2.1 Old Fourth Ward

This intown neighborhood is primarily a residential area of low-income apartments and boarding houses, with some businesses such as markets and the infamous (and now closed) Claremont Motor Inn and Lounge. Most residents are working-class African-Americans (AAs), although there has been a gentrification movement over the last 3 years to attract homeowners of higher incomes, including both young AA and White professionals. The most prevalent drugs are marijuana and crack cocaine, with some heroin use on the southern side near Cabbagetown. There are a significant number of professional sex workers. The area includes Sweet Auburn and Edgewood Avenue, communities that originally housed workers at a nearby mill in Cabbagetown and their families. African-Americans living in the Fourth Ward worked the second and third shifts at the mill.

5.2.2.2 Mechanicsville

The residents in this old, industrial neighborhood immediately south of downtown are mainly low-income and AA. A lack of jobs and substandard housing are chronic problems in this neighborhood. Jobs were historically industrial and related to the nearby railroad, or based on city services. The most prevalent drugs are crack-cocaine and heroin, the latter being concentrated for the past several decades on three blocks of Smith Street, a street which has been the focus of an intensive residential gentrification program coinciding with the 1996 Summer Olympic games and the Empowerment Zone funds.

The three peripheral communities related to the study were Cabbagetown, English Avenue/Vine City, and several Southwest Atlanta neighborhoods.

5.2.2.3 Cabbagetown

The intown neighborhood immediately south of the Old Fourth Ward and north of Grant and Ormewood Parks is primarily residential and primarily populated by low-income Whites who moved to Atlanta from the north Georgia Appalachian Mountains. The most prevalent drugs are crack-cocaine, heroin, and methamphetamine. There are significant numbers of sex workers in the neighborhood. The neighborhood residents have historically been considered very hostile toward AAs. The community was originally based on working the first shift at the Atlanta Bag and Cotton Mill. Recently, the mill (which closed in 1970) has been converted into up-scale studio apartments and serves as a basis for gentrification of the entire neighborhood.

5.2.2.4 English Ave/Vine City

These neighborhoods make up a semimythical area of town referred to by heroin users as "The Bluff." The term is not place-specific, but describes the general locale for scoring high-quality heroin. The most prevalent drug by far is heroin, although crack-cocaine, marijuana, and methamphetamine are also obtainable. Owing to its proximity to social institutions such as Georgia Institute of Technology and Fulton County Jail, the area is quite varied although mainly residential. Lack of affordable housing combined with the lack of jobs and easy money to be made from drug work has destabilized the neighborhood, resulting in a visible number of "junkies" at all times of the day. In addition, nearby streets are noted for their high incidence of violent crimes. While these neighborhoods are also experiencing gentrification, they differ from other neighborhoods in that new building projects are primarily nonresidential in nature, such as the King Plough Art Center.

5.2.2.5 Southwest Atlanta

Generally referred to simply as the SWATs, this part of town is a sprawling area that incorporates several neighborhoods. A residential neighborhood, the SWATs combines middle-class homes with numerous public and low-income apartment complexes. Although the neighborhoods were relatively integrated up until about 25 years ago, the population in the area today is almost entirely AA, and joblessness and crime are increasing. The most prevalent drug in the area is marijuana, although both crack-cocaine and heroin can be obtained.

5.3 DATA COLLECTION

5.3.1 *Questionnaire design*

The Urban and Rural Networks Projects drew heavily on the instruments and approaches used in Colorado Springs (see Chapter 4). Some wording and question order was changed to acknowledge differences in community dialect. Also, the standard

NIDA drug ascertainment questionnaire was used instead of the format used in Colorado Springs. A brief "quiz" on HIV, which was included in Colorado Springs at the request of the funding agency (Center for Diseases Control and Prevention, CDC), was omitted in Flagstaff/Atlanta. But in general, investigators in Flagstaff/Atlanta attempted to collect all of the same demographic, historical, and behavioral variables. A similar approach was used to define and ascertain network partners (sexual, social, drug-using, and needle-sharing). Also, a "matrix" questionnaire, asking each respondent to describe the relationships between all pairs of partners, was adopted from the Colorado Springs study. Data layout and data processing were virtually identical among the studies, with only minor technical differences.

5.3.1.1 Name generators
In this study, as in its antecedents, names were generated by first asking persons to provide a list (with initials or other markers) of their main social partners (persons with whom they shared meals or rooms, or with whom they interacted daily), and all their sexual and drug-using or needle-sharing partners. In keeping with expectations, most relationships were multiplex (involving more than one of these relationships). No limit was placed on the number of partners that could be named, and although there were some very large lists, most persons' lists were less than 15 and averaged between 8 and 10 per respondent.

5.3.1.2 Survey instrument
The same instrument was used for the baseline and follow-up interviews, and the core set of questions was divided into five main sections: psychosocial and demographic; drug-related HIV risk; self-reported sexual behaviors; social network ascertainment; and a "matrix" section. Although the instrument included some explicit (and possibly embarrassing or uncomfortable) questions, respondents seemed willing to discuss their lifestyle decisions with very little prompting. These questionnaires were administered face-to-face, without use of computer aids (the study preceded the publication of data showing that ACASI was an effective method and might, in some populations, be superior to face-to-face interviews). In general, an interview took about 45 min to administer, though several hours to days may have been required in setting it up. The network section asked a series of questions about each of the contacts named (see Questionnaire) and contained a matrix section that asked the respondent to define the relationships that he or she knew about between each pair of contacts. The time required to administer this section was obviously a function of the number of contacts. Later stage interviews were substantially shorter since a considerable portion of the obtained information would have been unchanged, a 6-month period was evaluated instead of a lifetime, and respondents were habituated to the interview.

During the process of recruitment and interview preparation, a two-page "locator" was also developed for each participant. This provided information on the possible places that staff could find the respondent, and general information that would help in subsequent location attempts. These locators proved extremely useful in the follow-up of persons whose lives were chaotic and unpredictable.

5.3.2 Qualitative components

Considerable qualitative evaluation was required for this project to proceed. Unlike top–down surveys, network approaches use bottom up methods to build a picture of the community. Such an approach is obviously necessitated by the elusive nature of the persons at risk. A traditional sampling frame is highly likely to miss such persons. The project also faced a number of challenges in ascertaining the risk networks of chronic drug users in the study communities. As a result, the staff had to develop methods to address the variety of problems encountered. We describe their methods in some detail in subsequent sections.

5.3.3 Biological specimens

Participants were tested for HIV using the oral HIV test. (Orasure®). If the respondent was known to be HIV+, blood was also collected to assess $CD4^+$ counts.

5.4 FIELDWORK EXPERIENCES

In addition to the design issues that required ethnographic approaches (see Section 4), other problems encountered in the early months of the project provided several lessons for the conduct of these studies. The Principal Investigator (Rothenberg) had little experience working directly in the street with the communities at risk and thus had little basis for selecting appropriate staff. The original field interviewers, though highly competent, had concerns about safety that diminished their effectiveness in recruiting and interviewing. There was a high turnover in street outreach workers, a high level of staff conflict, and low morale. Several breakdowns in study continuity occurred because of staff conflicts. Certain verbal tics epitomized some of the attitudes that developed. Interviewers, for example, spoke of having to get respondents to "give up" their contacts. There was a negative attitude toward reimbursing clients for their time, perhaps related in part to the feeling that staff were being "hustled." By the end of the first 2 years, however, a gradual changeover in staff led to a better equilibrium and improved street outreach and interviewing. The study was thus completed with a stable and efficient group that has now been assigned similar activities on other projects.

5.4.1 Entrée into the field

To begin, we identified high intensity drug-using communities based on the experience of public health outreach workers and other drug researchers. The first activity in every community was to introduce ourselves to community members through the public health outreach practice of setting up an information table for 1 or 2 days in the proximity of an active drug and prostitution strip. During these times we passed out condoms, HIV literature, drinks and snacks, introduced ourselves to local community residents, and described the purposes and procedures of our project. Often one of our outreach workers recognized a member of the community who they knew from their earlier years "in the life" or from their work on other projects, which helped facilitate our entry to the community.

This initial activity generated subjects for the study and provided the ethnographer with candidates for open-ended interviews. These interviews involved life and drug use histories, and sex and drug network questions. They also provided knowledge and contacts for identifying representative network seeds and promoted rapport. As general social and drug use patterns began to emerge, male and female network seeds who met the necessary criteria were selected.

5.4.1.1 Initial network recruitment

Our first research site was a small intersection whose cross streets extended several blocks in all four directions with a few dilapidated houses, a junk yard/car repair site, and some open lots. Though the location was known as a primary site for "copping" heroin, drug quality was variable. Few of the injecting drug users (IDUs) who frequented the area lived in the vicinity, and it was only one of several sites that they frequented. Unpredictable police surveillance increased the difficulty of locating clients at this site for follow-up.

Our initial respondents presented networks of relatively small size, reporting only a few drug and sex partners. High levels of repeated, overlapping mentions of partners, and restricted or refused access to partners (e.g. fearful of disclosure of drug use to family or sex partners) compounded the often fleeting or absent presence of network members in the community. Furthermore, very few respondents gave full names or addresses of their partners, and many were regularly incarcerated.

In our first research community we conducted interviews with 15 people before selecting our first seed who filled the profile of a typical male drug user in the community. Our first seed was a 40 year old, male heroin and/or cocaine (speedball) IDU who was a regular partner of a local drug-using network in the community. However, after interviewing him, we found that his network only consisted of seven individuals. Three of these were female sex partners that he did not want us to contact because they were unaware of his drug use. We attempted to recruit four of his male drug-use network partners, but within 1 month of their identification, two of the partners were in jail and not available for interview. Soon thereafter, our seed was hospitalized with endocarditis. However, we had the seed select a network partner for the second node in the chain and did a full relational interview with him. This individual provided five network partners, although he too had only three partners available for interviews, and we were able to continue to develop the Chain Link network from this individual's partners. As this network developed it provided limited access to network partners and presented many dead-end relations, so that we could only develop it to seven steps.

5.4.1.2 Subsequent recruitment activity

This experience in our first community led us to develop strategies for accessing network partners and also to expand our criteria for identifying subsequent research communities. We realized that ensuring the confidentiality of all disclosed network partners' names and addresses, as well as their sex and drug risk behavior, was critical to collect valid information and secure the assistance of respondents in locating their partners. As mentioned, some respondents did not want their partners contacted; others did not know their partners' full names or whereabouts and some partners refused participation. When unable to enlist a partner or node we "reflected back" to the node from which this partner was identified and recruited another of this person's partners. When we reached a dead-end and the previous network had no available partners, we "returned to the origin," that is went back to the seed, selected another partner, and continued developing the network.

It was clear from the work in our first community that we needed a community with a large and localized population of drug users. Therefore, the second research community we chose, was one that had families of drug users living nearby, an open-air drug market, park and liquor house congregation sites, many sites for drug use and for users to live, and social services and commercial activities. As a result, drug users in the community were not as likely to disappear for months. Of course, as police activity and gentrification increased, the viability of local resources to support drug use began to wane.

We also learned from our early work that we needed a seed who was rooted in community drug use and subsistence, who had a substantial network that could be accessed for interviews and who would cooperate in recruiting his or her partners and introduce the project to them. It was also important to enlist male and female seeds who were part of different network enclaves so that there would not be an inordinate number of cross-links or shared partners. Otherwise we could have enlisted the links of a single, insular network that would miss much of the variation in community social and HIV risk behaviors and relations. In this way our findings reflected much of the network structure and dynamics of HIV drug and sex risk behavior in our research communities.

For our second community, we spent a good deal of time finding male and female drug users with these characteristics. As opposed to conducting fifteen interviews over three and a half weeks to find the first seed in our initial community, it took thirty-five interviews and 5 weeks to find our first seed in our second community. Preliminary ethnographic interviews allowed us to identify seeds with substantial networks whose members were relatively available.

Utilizing these criteria in community and seed selection facilitated our ability to complete subsequent networks. For instance, we were able to expand by 27 the number of respondents in the second Chain Link network and were able to complete ten steps in the network as opposed to seven in the first community. We also saw a 39 percent decrease in the number of respondents not available for interviews between the two communities. Moreover, although these networks were of markedly different sizes, the number of variations in the sequences of selecting partners ended up to be the same.

Also, in the face of repeatedly hard to locate respondents and questionable network information, we realized that a team effort would improve our ability to identify the networks and gather credible information. Therefore, we instituted daily outreach worker, interviewer, and project ethnographer meetings to share formal and informal information on network relations, notable drug or sex risk behavior and community events (e.g. police busts, violence). These debriefing and strategizing sessions improved our ability to locate hard-to-find network partners, identify erroneous or duplicate network partners, and validate or crosscheck individual and network risk behavior and relationships. It also provided a means to coordinate the identification and recruitment of isolates who expanded the range of information on network and community relations and behavior.

5.4.1.3 Field staff

The Atlanta group used multiple field teams to cover several research sites simultaneously. The field teams were composed of staff representing two types of professionals—interviewers and outreach workers—with distinct skills and responsibilities. Interviewers typically engaged in the formal aspects of the research, such as assessing potential respondents' eligibility to participate, scheduling respondents for follow-up interviews, ensuring informed consent, conducting the interview, checking the face validity of data, and distributing fees and incentives. All of the interviewers had at least some graduate-level education, as well as previous research experience. The outreach staff was engaged in accessing the research population. Outreach staff varied widely in terms of previous research experience (none to extensive) and education (GED to a bachelor's degree). The skills needed to perform outreach activities, however, are not based on formal training. Rather, they are gained through direct exposure to community life. The more important qualifications of all outreach staff were their extensive experience with street hustles (such as using and dealing drugs) and, for several, a history of incarceration.

5.4.2 Gatekeeper interactions

The objective of our outreach efforts was to penetrate aspects of the community, which are inherently "hard-to-reach." Barriers to research within this population derive from fear of official authority, such as the police, and the severe penalties associated with engaging in behaviors such as illicit drug use. Outreach staff were recruited from the communities themselves and provided with training pertinent to the goals of the research. As a result, the study was able to establish credibility within the research communities based on the reputation of the outreach staff, as well as their social links to community members. An essential issue to community penetration is negotiating the presence of *insidership*, usually communicated through familiarity with local culture. Once some level of insidership is established, status within the existing social hierarchy must be negotiated. Outreach staff had maintained high-status reputations while they were "in the life," and these reputations (and associated behavioral scripts and styles) were still considered valid in the context of their researcher role.

5.4.3 *Procedures*

The primary responsibilities for the outreach workers included direct daily contact with study participants and other important members of the community sites. An important aspect of the outreach role was to provide an initial face validity assessment of potential respondents to ensure that: (*a*) that they were who they said they were; (*b*) that they understood the purpose of the interview; and (*c*) that there would be no negative outcome from their reporting behaviors such as intravenous drug usage or homosexual sexual behaviors. Other outreach activities not directly related to the study included informing community members of the aims of the research project, providing information on local health and addiction services and programs, and distributing condoms.

Both male and female project staff had to manage social and sexual issues. Several members of the research team were young (early twenties to early forties), attractive AA women. They constantly had to negotiate how their appearance influenced their interaction with respondents. In particular, they had to set limits with romantically inclined respondents and diffuse hostilities among female community members who felt insecure or threatened by their presence. A related phenomenon occurred in the interactions between male staff and female respondents. Since a number of the respondents were women who engaged in the exchange of sex for money, they often perceived staff to be ideal solicitation candidates since they were (compared with the majority of men in the community sites) wealthy, healthy, respectful, and attentive. In contrast to the experiences of the female staff, overtures made to male staff were much more directly sexual in nature. During the interaction, male staff had to delicately set limits by acknowledging the overtures and refusing any offers without appearing condescending or "put off." One member of the research team was a young AA lesbian who was open about her sexuality and dressed in a stereotypical masculine (or "butch") fashion. Initial concerns of supervisory staff about her being the target of potential homophobia were unwarranted; she was extremely effective in reaching community members who were suspicious of the projects aims.

Maintaining daily field research activities at multiple sites requires a great deal of coordination and logistical preparation. To deal with this, we established a base-of-operations in the field using an apartment as a satellite interview locale. The office was located in a small apartment building approximately one block from a major crack-cocaine copping area that serviced the entire city. When respondents were unwilling or unable to be transported to the field office (usually as a result of time constraints during their hustle period, or simply their desire to maintain a watch on street activities/opportunities), interviews were conducted in a staff members' automobile, a relatively secluded outside location (such as a bench at the empty end of the park), or in the respondent's place of residence. In the latter circumstance, research staff were often presented with additional insights from observing activities during the interviews. These ranged from simple interruptions to actual risk-related behaviors. The field office also served as a means for respondents in the neighborhood to easily contact us with new information, or simply visit and talk with the staff members.

5.4.4 Incentives and motivation to participate

To motivate participation and follow-up, the project offered eligible respondents a $20 incentive. In addition, research staff could use their discretion in compensating nonrespondents who had significantly aided the research team in locating a respondent or convincing eligible community members to participate.

Within any 30-day period there were variations in the availability and willingness of respondents to be interviewed. Since many of the community members in the study received some form of government financial assistance, it was often difficult to locate or interview respondents immediately after the first of the month when their subsidy checks arrived (an event known in the street as "Mother's Day"). Some respondents had to take care of all their financial obligations such as rent and bills. For respondents who used illicit drugs, this was also a time for them to purchase large amounts of drugs and often rent a room if they did not have secure housing. Even for community members who did not directly receive any government subsidy, the influx of money into the neighborhood economy at the beginning of every month provided regular opportunities for personal profit. Usually by the beginning of the third week, however, most community members were low on funds and were looking for ways to supplement their income. Thus, the $20 research incentive became very attractive, and it became easier to locate respondents and interview them.

The monetary incentive became a point of contention in a variety of ways. Occasionally, some full-relational interview respondents would apparently bolster their social network contacts with two or three fictitious individuals identified only through the use of a pseudonym. Since the person was fictitious, the research team was dependent on the respondent to act as a gatekeeper, for which the respondent expected compensation. The respondent would make the description suitably ambiguous so that they could then locate a relatively obscure community member and prepare them to act as the fictitious contact. Follow-up with these "pseudo-respondents" became nearly impossible, and it was only after people could not remember their supposed close social contacts after six months that their deception became apparent and the hustle was revealed. By the second round of interviews, most of the respondents understood the basic logistics of the selection process and would develop arrangements to nominate other community members as a social contact for a fee. In some instances when the respondent had not had sufficient time to discuss the matter with a person they had nominated, they would attempt to intimidate or otherwise manipulate the nominee into sharing the incentive with them.

5.4.5 Confidentiality concerns

One problem that arose in the midst of the research was the belief shared by community members that we only interviewed people who were already HIV seropositive. The study started to be referred to as the "AIDS survey" since the protocol involved drawing blood for an HIV screening test and additional CD4 counts for respondents known to have already seroconverted. The research protocol actually focused much more on seronegative recruitment, but many individuals who had only had previous experience with health department personnel assumed that regular follow-up implied infection. Some respondents became uncomfortable associating with the research staff since they felt it gave them the reputation on the street as being positive. In at least two instances, respondents feared that research staff had violated their confidentiality or were intentionally giving community members the impression that they were diseased or dangerous.

Also, infrequently community members with whom the staff developed close relationships became unable to recognize staff's efforts as professionally motivated. This was particularly true for the Outreach staff who often shared similar life-histories with respondents or utilized the same community resources (e.g. NA/AA meetings, mutual friends and associates, etc.). The negative ramification of this was that at times respondents perceived (or attempted to manipulate staff by claiming to perceive) their confidentiality had been purposefully violated by staff sharing information with community members or spreading rumors. In addition, negative relationships among community members sometimes had an impact on their sentiments toward team members and the research. This was especially true when staff were present in the community for ethnographic or related reasons, but not directly engaged in interviewing.

In addition, the endemic presence of everyday prejudices and biases with regard to ethnicity, gender/sexuality, and HIV status, affected interaction among respondents and staff. The majority of our respondents (and members of the field site community in general) were mature, lower socioeconomic, AA men and women who had been raised in the South. In contrast, the research team was primarily composed of middle-class AAs (three males and nine females) and two White males. In street interactions, respondents often assumed that the white males were the senior staff who made the final decisions regarding selection of respondents and distribution of funds, when in actuality it was usually one of the AA female staff who made these decisions.

5.4.6 Interview strategies

In addition to the quantitative interview approach, ethnographic data were also collected using a qualitative interview. Respondents for these interviews were drawn from a nonrandom sample of those who had already been interviewed using the social network instrument. The purpose of the qualitative interview was to identify and assess the daily routines of network members, as articulated by themselves. Ethnographic data provided a more valid context by including detailed descriptions of activities and concerns related to daily life. Over the course of the study, research staff identified persons who held influential positions within multiple respondents' social networks, but who were never identified as contacts by respondents during baseline or follow-up. Typically of these "isolate" contacts were the suppliers of illicit services within the field site communities (such as running a house that supplied drugs, prostitutes, or illegal liquor), and respondents were hesitant to identify them for fear of jeopardizing their relationship (and by extension, their access to illicit services). In an attempt to assess the importance of such unnamed contacts, staff used an independent recruitment strategy wherein a single interview (i.e. baseline but no follow-up interviews) was conducted to incorporate the perspective of these unnamed "isolate" contacts.

5.4.7 Community-based partial network designs

Despite their urban facade, many community members defined their relevant social space narrowly. Although Atlanta is a city with nearly four million residents, most respondents in this study often did not leave their immediate neighborhoods. In one extreme example, a respondent had not left a half-mile radius from his home in over 2 years. From a field perspective, this immobility produces social network relations that appear complex and dense, similar to what one might expect to encounter in a rural village-like community.

From the turmoil of the earlier years and subsequent stabilization we learned several things. First, a long learning curve is required to assemble a field team that can work together and that has the right combination of street experience and academic background to be effective. Second, sufficient time must be built into studies that take place in the community to establish a knowledge and experience base for the field team. The trust and confidence of the community is vital to a study's success, and such trust is only earned through on-the-scene presence over a sufficiently long period of time. Third, though persons are paid for their time and cooperation, a field project of this type must provide something more to participants (in our case, condoms, drug treatment referral, and a variety of small favors, short of actually giving people money). Finally, a continuing reappraisal of the interview instrument and procedures is critical to the collection of dependable information, particularly in the face of personnel turnover.

5.5 ILLUSTRATIVE FINDINGS

The Urban Networks study collected 242 epidemiologic and demographic variables, as well as information on social network contacts and a matrix of interaction among all possible pairs of contacts. The epidemiological elements included information on general social circumstances (housing, sources of income), past medical history, past STD/HIV history, assessment of HIV risk, current drug activity (using the detailed NIDA questionnaire), and current sexual activity. Recurring interviews with persons in the networks permitted description of both stationary characteristics (gender, ethnicity) and changing characteristics (type of residence, source of income). Risk taking behavior was reported in both the general (*How often do you share needles with others?*) and the particular (*For a person named as a contact: Did you share needles with this person?*).

For each of the six community chains, we calculated basic networks characteristics for each of six groupings (all risks, sexual contact, drug-sharing, needle-sharing, social contact, and needle-sharing plus sexual contact) for each of three sets of interviews

Box 5.1. *Network Structure Features*

Size
Density
Transitivity
Centralization
    Degree centralization
    Closeness centralization
    Betweenness centralization
Information
Bonacich power
Components
    Largest component size
    K-cores
    Cliques ($n = 3, 4, 5$)
    2-Cliques ($n = 3$)
    2-plex ($n = 3, 4, 5$)
Concurrency (κ_3)

(the frequency of interviews four, five, and six was insufficient to warrant separate analyses), for a total of 108 networks. In addition to visualization using KRACKPLOT (available at www.contrib.andrew.cmu.edu/~krack), we used UCINet-V (Borgatti et al. 1999) to calculate a standard set of network statistics (see Box 5.1).

The measure of concurrency, described by Morris and Kretzchmar (1995), was calculated directly from the mean degree and variance of each network. As appropriate, network variables that relate to individuals (e.g. degree, closeness, betweenness) or network variables that relate to the network in which the individual is found (e.g. density, components, microstructures, concurrency) were analyzed together with epidemiological variables. Mixing matrices based on age, gender, ethnicity, level of sexual activity, and numerous other characteristics were also available from these data.

The matrix interview provided interesting information that can be incorporated into the original graph of a community chain. In general, matrix information increases the number of edges in a graph by 1.5–2 times. It is uncertain, however, how valid this information is. As part of a supplement to this project, we collected information on 275 additional persons using a snowball design that began with five different "seeds." The snowball permitted direct comparison of information obtained by the matrix approach with information provided by contacts. This supplemental study interviewed each participant only once, but used the same instruments and approach.

5.5.1 Enrollment

In Atlanta, the six original chains contained 157 respondents who identified a total 1253 contacts during their first interview. During subsequent interviews, new contacts were incorporated into the sampling plan, and those interviewed during the first wave, but not named subsequently were reinterviewed. In all, 228 persons were included in the interviews in the community chains. In addition, a number of persons felt to be ethnographically important were interviewed, though not included as part of the community chains ("isolates"), bringing the total number of persons enrolled in the study to 293, and the total number of contacts named to 4500. In Flagstaff, a difference in interpretation of the study design produced a somewhat different configuration. Though the original intent may have been to keep the six community chains mutually exclusive (in terms of respondents), field interviewers found it difficult to do so in the smaller environment of Flagstaff. Thus, ninety-five persons were originally enrolled into the six chains, but many of them belonged to more than one chain. These ninety-five persons occupied 157 positions within the chains. In all, they named 504 different contacts during their initial interview. An additional 159 persons, not part of these six chains, who formed small additional groupings, were also interviewed (analogous to the "isolates" in Atlanta).

As noted, since this discussion originates from the Atlanta group, it will focus more on the events and findings from Atlanta.

5.5.2 Follow-up

As noted, 293 persons were recruited into the study. Of these 228 were members of the six community chains, and the remainder were "isolates." Of the 228 members, 157 were part of the original recruitment into the six chains. Additional persons were added during subsequent interviews, as new contacts were named by respondents. There were 157 original interviews, 133 interviews in the second wave (85 percent), 122 in the third (77 percent), and 110 in the fourth (70 percent). These percentages are inflated, however, by the new persons added at each wave. Among the 157 persons who were first interviewed, 119 (76 percent) were interviewed at least twice and 90 (57 percent) were interviewed a third time. Among the entire group of 228 participants, 72 percent were interviewed at least twice.

5.5.3 Demographics, prevalence, and incidence

Within the six community chains, 62 percent of respondents were men and 38 percent were women. Eighty-nine percent of the overall group was AA, and 91 percent of all participants were over the age of thirty.

In the overall group, 234 (81 percent) persons were tested for HIV, and 31 (13.3 percent) were positive. Three seroconversions were observed during 164.8 person-years of observation, for an annualized incidence density of 1.8 percent. The calculated mean duration of infection in these circumstances was 7.4 years, and was consistent with the observed distribution of $CD4^+$ counts among infected persons (see Fig. 5.2). Fewer than 5 percent of HIV+ persons in this study had a $CD4^+$ count below $200/ml^3$.

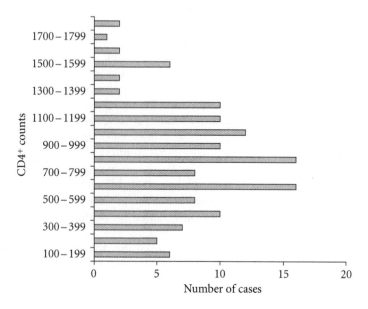

Figure 5.2. *Distribution of CD4⁺ Counts Urban Networks Study, Atlanta, GA 1995–9*

Table 5.1. *Distribution of Prevalence by Site and Type of Ascertainment*

Sample	First interview		Second interview		Third interview	
	N	%	*N*	%	*N*	%
Chain link						
Sites						
A	10	20.0	7	0.0	7	14.3
B	36	16.7	33	12.1	31	16.1
C	25	12.0	10	10.0	9	0.0
Random walk						
Sites						
A	23	8.7	20	10.0	23	13.0
B	31	12.9	22	13.6	18	11.1
C	32	12.5	41	9.8	24	4.2

Source: Urban Networks Study, Atlanta, GA 1995–9.

The prevalence of HIV-positivity differed markedly by site, interview, and method of ascertainment (Table 5.1). No HIV-positive person was detected within the Chain Link group during the second round of interviews at site A. In contrast, the prevalence at this site during the first interview was 20 percent and was 14.3 percent during the third interview. The remarkable changeover in composition of the group over this 18-month period attests to the volatile nature of the groups of at-risk persons. Such variation, somewhat less dramatic, was observed at site C as well. On the other hand, results from site B were relatively uniform. Taken together, these observations suggest a moving network target whose specific relationship to risk may be difficult to quantify.

5.5.4 Distribution of risk

Similarly, there was considerable diversity in the prevalence of risky behaviors through the six community chains (Table 5.2). The proportion of needle-sharing contacts varied from 5.2 percent (site B, third interview, Chain Link) to 57.4 percent (site A, first interview Chain Link). The variation in sexual contacts was smaller, though the proportion in different subsets varied by more than two-fold. In addition to the diversity of risk, the distribution of contacts demonstrates the high level of risk in which persons in these communities actually engaged. Such observations are in qualitative agreement with the amount and type of risk that persons told us they generally engaged in.

5.5.4.1 Drug risk

In general, HIV+ and HIV− persons did not differ markedly in their drug-use behavior (data on specific drug use are voluminous and will not be shown here; see appended survey instrument). HIV+ women tended to inject more than HIV− women, but overall, the HIV− group had more needle exposure and more needle-sharing (Table 5.3). The high level of needle activity among HIV+ persons was due in part to several injectors whose needle use was intense and unrelenting

Table 5.2. *Distribution of Sexual and Needle-Sharing Contacts, by Site, Interview, and Type of Network Ascertainment*

	First interview			Second interview			Third interview		
	N	Sexual (%)	Needle (%)	N	Sexual (%)	Needle (%)	N	Sexual (%)	Needle (%)
Chain link Sites									
A	61	16.4	57.4	89	15.7	23.6	40	22.5	60.0
B	271	33.2	22.5	167	31.7	12.6	155	19.4	5.2
C	157	21.0	28.0	42	31.0	14.3	38	39.5	15.8
Random walk Sites									
A	224	19.6	21.9	132	20.5	6.1	157	18.5	11.5
B	254	23.2	15.0	181	18.8	0.0	94	20.2	4.3
C	206	30.6	9.7	214	26.2	10.7	97	29.9	4.1

Source: Urban Networks Study, Atlanta, GA 1995–9.

Table 5.3. *Comparison of Needle Use in HIV-Positive and HIV-Negative Persons*

| Total Cohort = 292 | Total Tested for HIV = 234 (81%) | |
	HIV-positive	HIV-negative
Number	31	203
Active Drug Users[a]	8 (25.8%)	47 (23.2%)
Average daily exposure to injections		
Entire group[b]	2.0 injections/day	2.4 injections/day
Injectors	7.8 injections/day	10.3 injections/day

[a] Defined as persons who injected drugs during the previous 3 months.
[b] Defined as the proportion of days injected during the month times the average number of injections per day among those who inject drugs.

Source: Urban Networks Study, Atlanta, GA 1995–9.

despite infection. The amount of needle prophylaxis was the same in both HIV+ and HIV− persons. Between 50 and 75 of persons (by gender) stated that they had cleaned their works with bleach in the last 30 days. Roughly 25 percent of both groups had shared needles in the last 90 days (data not shown).

5.5.4.2 Sexual risk
The level of reported sexual risk-taking was high, but not substantially different for HIV+ and HIV− persons. Nearly 30 percent of both positive and negative men, for example, practiced insertive anal intercourse, and, on average, about half the respondents reporting having sex with an IDU. Sixty percent of the HIV+ men reported continuing receptive anal exposure (Table 5.4). Similarly, condom use did not differ substantially by gender and HIV status, with the notable exception that HIV+ women reported a high use of condoms for vaginal sex. The overall reported level of condom use for vaginal sex was between 50 and 60 percent and substantially lower for oral and anal sex (Table 5.5).

5.5.5 Comparison of Atlanta and Flagstaff

Using results from the first interview, some comparisons of risk taking at the two sites can be made (Table 5.6). In Atlanta, the levels of homelessness, less than a high school education, and unemployment are close to 50 percent. Ten percent of the women in Atlanta stated that they worked as prostitutes, though far higher proportions indicated that they had exchanged sex for drugs or money. Drug use patterns at the two sites were markedly different, particularly with regard to the frequent use of crack-cocaine and the injection of heroin or cocaine in Atlanta and the use of amphetamines and marijuana in Flagstaff. Similarly, the level of sexual risk (number of partners; sex with an IDU) in Atlanta was considerably greater than that in Flagstaff. Interestingly, however, the level of prophylactic behavior (cleaning needles, condom use), though low in both areas, was higher in Atlanta. Forty percent of persons in Atlanta felt that

Table 5.4. *Sexual Risks by Sex and HIV Status*

	HIV-positive		HIV-negative	
	Men	Women	Men	Women
Sex with men (%)	22	100	7	98
Sex with women (%)	89	23	99	35
Sex with an injecting drug user	65	54	49	43
Given money for sex	47	0	62	16
Given drugs for sex	71	0	73	22
Received money for sex	29	77	32	73
Received drugs for sex	35	69	30	58
Insertive anal intercourse	29	0	26	0
Receptive anal intercourse	60	15	2	17

Source: Urban Networks Study, Atlanta, GA 1995–9.

Table 5.5. *Reported Condom Use*

	HIV-positive		HIV-negative	
	Men ($N=18$)	Women ($N=13$)	Men ($N=143$)	Women ($N=116$)
Oral sex	39.2	64.2	20.6	39.2
Anal sex	15.8	8.3	12.8	5.0
Vaginal sex	57.9	83.3	53.2	64.2

Source: Urban Networks Study, Atlanta, GA 1995–9.

Table 5.6. *Comparison of Findings: Atlanta and Flagstaff (First Interview Data)*

Variable	Atlanta	Flagstaff
Education, employment, income		
Dropped out of high school	52.3	39.9
Homeless	40.4	10.6
Unemployed	54.4	35.6
Works as prostitute	10.2	0.4
Works as drug dealer	1.0	0.0
Source of income: paying job[a]	36.1	53.7
Source of income: welfare[a]	37.5	35.0
Source of income: other person[a]	62.8	65.6
General personal risk status		
Has changed habits because of HIV	83.7	73.9
Personal chances of getting HIV (high or medium)	41.3	25.9
Ever given drugs for sex	45.9	5.2
Ever given money for sex	37.1	3.1

Table 5.6. (*Continued*)

Variable	Atlanta	Flagstaff
Ever received drugs for sex	46.6	10.0
Ever received money for sex	53.9	10.9
Know anyone with HIV	85.0	60.8
Chance of others you know having HIV (high or medium)	76.2	64.2
Drug-taking and sexual risks		
Used alcohol in the last 6 months	85.9	87.6
Used Marijuana in the last 6 months	57.3	70.0
Used Crack in the last 6 months	79.6	42.9
Used Cocaine in the last 6 months	30.6	27.0
Used Heroin in the last 6 months	20.9	9.0
Used Heroin/Cocaine (speedball) in the last 6 months	16.5	6.4
Used Methadone in the last 6 months	5.8	5.5
Used opiates in the last 6 months	7.8	9.4
Used amphetamines in the last 6 months	2.4	38.2
Injected Cocaine in the last 30 days	24.3	8.6
Injected Heroin in the last 30 days	17.0	8.2
Injected Heroin/Cocaine in the last 30 days	14.6	4.7
Injected Methadone in the last 30 days	1.0	0.4
Injected opiates in the last 30 days	1.5	1.7
Injected amphetamines in the last 30 days	1.0	9.9
No. of days injected Cocaine in the last 30 days[b]	5.5 (0–30)	1 (0–20)
No. of days injected Heroin in the last 30 days[b]	4.5 (0–30)	3 (0–30)
No. of days injected Heroin/Cocaine in the last 30 days[b]	20 (0–30)	1 (0–15)
No. of days injected Methadone in the last 30 days[b]	0 (0–0)	0 (0–5)
No. of days injected opiates in the last 30 days[b]	0 (0–15)	0 (0–1)
No. of days injected amphetamines in the last 30 days[b]	0 (0–2)	0 (0–25)
Ever shared works with others	20.9	9.9
Shared in the last 30 days	6.8	3.9
Cleaned works after the last time they were used	17.0	10.3
Cleaned works with bleach	22.8	10.7
Sexual preference	87.9	89.7
Use condom for anal sex	9.6	1.3
Use condom for oral sex	30.8	0.9
Use condom for vaginal sex	59.2	2.5
Had sex with IDU	45.6	31.8
No. of sex partners in the past 30 days[b]	2 (0–450)	1 (0–30)
No. of sex partners in the past 6 months[b]	3 (0–2700)	1 (0–59)

[a] Sources of income are not mutually exclusive.
[b] Median (Range). All other values are percentages.

they were at significant risk of contracting HIV/AIDS; only 25 percent of those in Flagstaff thought so. (In an interesting comparison, about 28 percent of persons over-all in Colorado Springs felt themselves to be at high risk. In view of the existing prevalence in these three communities, these assessments may be on the mark.)

5.5.5.1 Network structure

The 108 different network configurations provide considerable detail on network structure and change. Preliminary analyses indicate, however, that these observations may not form convenient or consistent patterns (Table 5.7). For example, the data associated with the multiplex networks of people who shared needles or had sex together display several interesting patterns but no clear direction. In general, components increased in number over the study period. However, there were several exceptions, indicating ongoing segmentation with possible reassembly. Degree varied from about 1.5 to 2.0 during the three interviews, while kappa, a measure of concurrency, showed a more consistent pattern of decrease during the interval. Other measures of the amount of structure (the last five columns of Table 5.7) were generally stable or decreasing (see, for example, the structure called "2-plex ($n = 3$)," which represents an open triad). Higher order structures (e.g. 4-cliques) were notably absent.

The three observed seroconversions took place in a setting of multiplex risk. Two occurred at Site A (Chain Link) and one at Site B (Chain Link). These groupings do not immediately stand out as having singular properties, and the number of outcomes is too few to warrant a multivariate approach. Nonetheless, it might be broached that the presence of only moderate structural elements, declining concurrency and increasing fragmentation as is suggested by these networks is consistent with a moderate level of endemic transmission. The relative constancy of personal risk-taking over the period of observation (data shown only for the first interview), at a level usually assumed to be significant for continuing transmission, suggests that the lack of structural change is a critical factor in preventing higher level endemic transmission. A stronger basis for this hypothesis awaits more detailed analyses of all the available network groupings, and the simultaneous consideration of network and behavioral change. In the absence of a significant number of outcomes, these data are unlikely to provide direct evidence of the relative role of behavioral and structural variables, but may provide indirect support of the relative importance of structural dynamics.

5.6 SOME METHODOLOGICAL ISSUES

Network analysis of this type of data poses several important challenges. First, it is a given that there are missing links, but that their characteristics and placement are not known. The use of matrix information provides added information, but its value has not been fully confirmed. Modeling the existence of additional links, based on the frequency and characteristics of known links, may be an acceptable approach, but requires appropriate variance inflation, or perhaps the use of a Monte Carlo technique that calculates network characteristics using a set of assumptions. The advantage of this technique is that it places the observed information in a context of the reasonable range of network characteristics from which the observed sample may have been drawn.

Second, networks vary considerably in size, as is evident from the data presented here, and certain network measures are size dependent. For example, density (usually calculated as observed edges/potential edges) will decrease as a function of the square of the number of nodes. The number of microstructures will increase with the

Table 5.7. *Network Characteristics for Network Groupings that Include Sexual or Needle-Sharing Associations*

Site	Type	Int.	Number	Density	Components	Degree	Kappa	Information	Clique (n = 3)	Clique (n = 4)	2-Clique (n = 3)	2-Plex (n = 3)	2-Plex (n = 4)
A	CL	1	33	0.038	2	2.18	9.62	0.462	2	1	8	135	4
		2	29	0.037	3	1.93	6.93	0.470	2	0	5	92	0
		3	33	0.028	3	1.82	3.78	0.567	0	0	4	179	0
A	RW	1	87	0.012	9	1.98	4.54	0.497	5	0	21	354	10
		2	48	0.015	16	1.33	1.67	1.130	0	0	8	27	0
		3	45	0.024	6	2.04	2.96	0.603	7	0	13	135	6
B	CL	1	116	0.009	6	1.98	6.23	0.355	2	0	31	411	2
		2	72	0.012	12	1.67	3.76	0.496	0	0	16	160	0
		3	51	0.013	17	1.33	1.66	1.090	0	0	6	46	0
B	RW	1	94	0.010	9	1.89	6.24	0.418	2	0	19	334	1
		2	48	0.015	15	1.38	1.26	1.060	0	0	14	23	0
		3	31	0.024	10	1.36	1.22	1.050	0	0	6	20	0
C	CL	1	68	0.015	7	1.85	5.08	0.449	1	0	14	210	1
		2	25	0.030	8	1.36	2.67	1.160	0	0	5	19	0
		3	32	0.023	9	1.44	0.45	0.996	0	0	4	45	0
C	RW	1	89	0.010	16	1.66	3.27	0.597	0	0	19	171	1
		2	92	0.008	25	1.48	3.86	0.886	1	0	13	161	0
		3	63	0.012	16	1.49	4.35	0.881	0	0	13	105	0

Notes: A, B, and C refer to the three community sites; RW = Random walk; CL = Chain link.
Kappa is defined as a function of the mean and variance of the degree: $(\sigma^2/\mu) + \mu - 1$; it is calculated only for respondents, and does not include contacts who were not interviewed.
Number refers to the number of persons (respondents plus contacts) in a given network configuration.
Degree is the number of direct connections to each person in the graph. *Information* is a centrality measure that computes the average distance from any person to all other persons in a connected component. A *Clique* of size *n* is a group of *n* persons all of whom are connected to each other. An *N-Clique* of size *n* is a group of *n* persons, each of whom is at least *N* steps from every other person in the grouping. A *k-plex* (*n*) is a group wherein every member is at least *n* − *k* steps from every other member. See text for discussion of density and component.

Source: Urban Networks Study, Atlanta, GA 1995–9.

size of the network, and thus render comparison of "the amount of structure" moot. Some measures, such as kappa (defined as the mean number of concurrent relationships per relationship) may be sensitive to network size because of the availability of partners for concurrency. In these data, kappa, calculated for all 108 networks, has a distinct relationship to network size (Fig. 5.3).

Third, one of the potential functions of this type of analysis is to predict which persons will become infected, and in which groups. Being able to identify the persons at highest risk for seroconversion, or for acquisition of an STD, has important preventive implications. In a multivariate construct that would include behavioral and network factors, the confidence limits for individual prediction are substantially larger than those for population prediction. This type of approach may thus be of value at the population level, but is unlikely to be of help at the individual level. The three seroconverters in this study (whose complete description was not included) exemplify this: it would have been difficult to single out these three.

Fourth, as is the case in this study, the small number of outcomes inhibits multivariate approaches that seek to examine the relative contribution of behavioral and network variables. In view of the expected (and realized) prevalence of 10–15 percent, a lower level of endemic transmission was observed than expected at the start of this study. Such "real world" observations impede validation of theoretical results from modeling that have significant implications both for understanding transmission and the development of interventions.

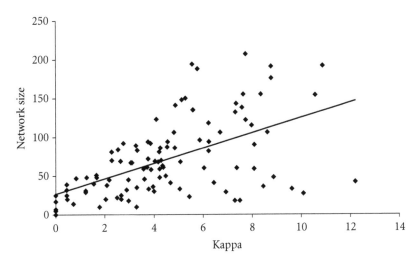

Figure 5.3. *Comparison of Network Size and Kappa in 108 Networks, Urban Networks Study, Atlanta, GA*

Notes: *Kappa* is defined as the proportion of contacts that are concurrent and may be calculated as a function of the mean and variance of the degree: $(\sigma^2/\mu) + \mu - 1$; it is calculated only for respondents, and does not include contacts who were not interviewed.

These challenges contribute to the agenda for further development of network approaches to transmission dynamics, and we hope to pursue them with data from this project and others. For this project specifically, we will continue the descriptive and analytic approaches outlined above, including calculation of risk configurations, stability indices, the joint distribution of behavioral factors and network features, more detailed comparisons of specific chains within sites, as well as comparison of the results from the two cities.

5.7 CONCLUSIONS

Network studies are difficult to perform, particularly when their focus is a serious illness and their content includes illicit or stigmatized behaviors. Work with populations at high risk for HIV and other conditions require considerable preparation, a long-term field presence, and the acquisition and training of qualified staff. The quality of information has a crucial relationship to the quality of interactions with the community, and results are easily distorted by inattention to the details of these interactions. In addition, the changing epidemiologic and ethnographic circumstances of a target area can make interpretation difficult. An observed change in network configuration can result from inappropriate positioning of research staff, from poor communication with participants, or from unsuspected ethnographic or environmental change.

With these caveats, we conclude that the network structure found in this study—fragmentation and lack of significant microstructure—fits theoretically with an environment that does not support rapid endemic transmission of HIV. Observations in areas of different prevalence are supportive, but do not provide direct quantitative links. This population demonstrates neither the intense needle-sharing that was evident in New York City during the late 1980s and early 1990s, nor the intense same-sex sexual activity that characterized the early years of the AIDS epidemic. This study suggests that a significant level of interactive needle-sharing, other drug use, heterosexual, and same sex risk may be needed to support endemic transmission in urban inner-city environments. Such an environment may ultimately constitute the major pattern for endemic transmission in industrialized countries.

References

Borgatti, S., Everett, M. et al. (1999). *UCINET 5.0 Version 1.00 for Windows: Software for Social Network Analysis*. Harvard, MA: Natick Analytic Technologies.

Morris, M. and Kretzschmar M. (1995). "Concurrent partnerships and transmission dynamics in networks," *Soc Net*, 17: 299–318.

6

The Seattle "Sexual Mixing," "Sexual Networks," and "Sexual Partnership Types" Studies

SEVGI O. ARAL, JIM HUGHES, PAMINA GORBACH, BRADLEY
STONER, LISA MANHART, GEOFF GARNETT, BETSY FOXMAN,
MATTHEW GOLDEN, AND KING K. HOLMES

6.1 INTRODUCTION

Sexually transmitted diseases (STDs) constitute a major disease burden globally (Aral et al. 1999). During the past three decades research attention has been focused on the contribution of sexual behaviors to the STD burden in a variety of social settings.

Several studies have failed to identify individual behavioral risk factors for STD; (Zenilman et al. 1988; Taha et al. 1996; Burstein et al. 1998; Ryan et al. 1998; Sturm et al. 1998). Although significant associations can usually be found, they seldom account for a large attributable risk of STD. Thus, not only the individual behaviors themselves, but also the specific epidemiologic and social contexts of the behaviors determine STD transmission (Aral et al. 1996). One important aspect of the epidemiologic context is the phase of the STD epidemic, reflected by the changing levels of prevalence of STD in specific subpopulations (Wasserheit and Aral 1996).

While measurement of individual sexual and other risk behaviors has improved remarkably in recent years (Turner et al. 1998), the study of the contexts in which these behaviors occur has advanced more slowly. Public health research approaches must move away from "individualization" of risk to the broader determinants of risk and disease (Padian et al. 1996; Diez-Roux 1998).

During the past decade, in a number of studies conducted in Seattle, Washington, we focused on aspects of social context associated with risk of acquiring or transmitting STD. More specifically we studied patterns of sexual mixing and sexual networks, and types of sexual partnerships, and described the associations between these parameters and STD risk.

6.2 SEXUAL MIXING PATTERNS AND STD: CONCEPTUAL FRAMEWORK

Sexual mixing patterns, broadly defined, refer to the partnership and network characteristics important to the spread of STD. A schematic rendering of our conceptual framework is presented in Fig. 6.1.

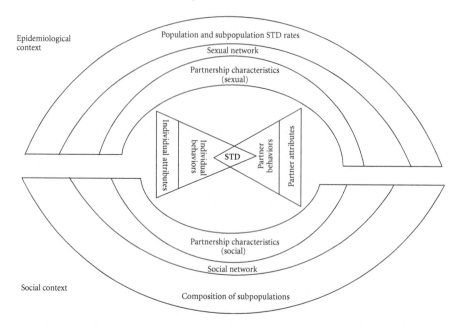

Figure 6.1. *Conceptual Framework of Mixing and STD Acquisition*

Note: The term mixing is meant here to encompass all interactions of the individual with partner in the context of networks and the community.

Here, individual STD status is located at the center of the figure, as the product of multiple layers of influence. The most proximate determinants of disease are the behaviors of an individual and his or her partner. Particular behaviors have different implications for different diseases; we focus on the behaviors most associated with gonorrhea, chlamydia, and human papilloma virus. The most neglected aspect of mixing and STD risk concerns the characteristics of sexual partners. Beyond behaviors, demographic attributes of individuals and their partners (such as age and ethnicity) offer an initial context in which partnerships are formed, and exert important influence on individual and partnership behaviors (Sonenstein et al. 1998). The next layer of influence is the partnership itself. Our work examines how both the social and sexual dimension of partnerships influence behaviors associated with STD risk. Sexual behaviors vary across partnership type in ways that could guide development of innovative and effective intervention strategies oriented toward high-risk partnerships.

At the next level, partnerships themselves may be embedded into networks of sexual contacts and social relationships. Social networks transmit social values and norms; it is important to understand the extent to which sexual networks are connected to broader social worlds. Our work focuses on the nature of overlap between sexual partnership types and social networks, and the effectiveness of local social control (exercised through social networks) over sexual risk taking. Finally, all of this occurs in specific epidemiological and social contexts. For example, structural factors, such as the demographic composition of the local population and the phase of the STD epidemic in subpopulations, determine the likelihood of acquisition of infection, given certain behaviors, and condition the structure of the social network, as well as opportunities for the formation of sexual partnerships.

6.2.1 Implications of mixing for disease burden, spread dynamics, and prevention

While patterns of social and sexual mixing, and the relationship between these two types of mixing are sociologically inherently interesting, the public health perspective requires definition of the role and relative importance of these parameters in determining the burden of disease, in informing prevention strategies, and in influencing diffusion of preventive interventions. Our studies have attempted to define the relative importance of sexual mixing in determining the disease burden in high and low disease prevalence subpopulations (Aral et al. 1999). Theoretical studies and other empirical studies of how specific patterns of sexual mixing influence disease burden will facilitate assessment of the potential impact of changes in sexual mixing patterns and related implications for prevention efforts.

Epidemiologists have exploited the concept of sexual mixing to develop a family of models that have been used to estimate the diffusion of STD. Initially, such models have relied on estimates of the rate of mixing between high- and low-risk populations, since collecting useable data on the sexual contact networks of individuals and populations is exceedingly difficult. We know that among the general population of adults: (*a*) there is a tendency toward "homophily" (in terms of basic sociodemographic characteristics) in partner selection (Laumann et al. 1994; Morris and Dean 1994; Joyner et al. 1998; Bearman et al. 2003); and (*b*) many adults recruit relationship partners from within their social networks (Laumann et al. 1994). Epidemiological research on STD, however, has revealed that people with STD tend to be "heavy mixers" meaning they have sex with two or more partners outside of their own social strata (Catania et al. 1995). This suggests that such partnerships may be discordant. Discordant pairs, characterized as representing links across social networks, may be responsible for the spread of STD between clusters in networks (Potterat et al. 1985). In one study of syphilis in North Carolina, partners of people with STD were not only often nonmonogamous, but were drawn from outside of the social network of the index patient, and were likely to be involved in exchange of sex for drugs (Thomas et al. 1995). The relational dynamics of socially or demographically discordant sexual dyads may differ from those of concordant dyads, affecting the communication within the partnership and issues of power and control, potentially important determinants of risky sexual behavior such as nonuse of condoms within a partnership. Epidemiological attention has been focused on the prevalence of non-homophilous, or discordant partnerships (e.g. partners not matched on age, race, geography, or social class background), because these partnerships—likely to act as functional bridges between otherwise unconnected populations—may serve as an important conduit for the spread of infection (Aral et al. 1999).

The National Health and Social Life Survey (NHSLS, see Chapter 1, this volume) described sexual mixing patterns in the United States based on a nationally representative sample of the general population, and related these to self reported history of STD (Laumann et al. 1994). Some investigations have focused on the influence of patterns of spatial mixing on the epidemiology of gonorrhea (Rothenberg 1983; Garnett and Anderson 1993). Others have explored patterns of mixing between groups with different levels of sexual activity (Hsu Schmitz and Castillo-Chavez 1994; Granath et al. 1991; Garnett et al. 1996), or between different age groups (Service and Blower 1995, 1996).

More recently, empirical studies of mixing patterns have demonstrated that specific patterns of mixing are indeed associated with increased risk for HIV infection (Service and Blower 1995, 1996), chlamydial infection (Aral et al. 1998), and gonorrhea (Aral et al. 1999). Many remaining knowledge gaps of particular, immediate concern involve both theoretical and analytical issues. For example, information is needed on why people mix in observed patterns; whether and how particular types of mixing are associated with particular attributes and types of partnerships; and on how perceptions and conceptualizations of the persons engaged in the partnerships and the mixing patterns mediate the associations between mixing patterns and attributes/types of partnerships.

Issues of measurement and analysis central to this field of investigation and still under development include definition and measurement of partnership, use of alternative potential approaches to analysis of sexual mixing (e.g. with the magnitude of attribute concordance between partners as the outcome variable; with the partnership as the unit of analysis; with the individual as the unit of analysis; etc.), and analysis of disease burden (e.g. in subpopulations defined by prevalence or demographic attributes).

In this chapter we present a number of specific questions on a variety of the subjects mentioned above and discuss the methodological approaches employed in attempting to answer the questions and summarize our findings. We also discuss the difficult issues in conceptualization, data collection and analysis, and ongoing work.

6.3 DESIGN OF THE SEATTLE DATA SETS

Starting in the early 1990s, studies on sexual mixing patterns, sexual networks, and sexual partnership types in Seattle were developed in several stages. Quantitative data were collected in surveys of Seattle populations with and without STD including sex partners of individuals with STD. Following analyses of these data, qualitative studies were undertaken to examine perceptions of partnership types and motivations for partnerships. The populations covered included attendees at STD clinics, attendees at non-STD health facilities, partners of STD-infected individuals reached through contact tracing, respondents recruited at sociogeographically specified areas of the city, and representative samples of the general population based on census tract of residence. Thus, subjects in our studies include random samples of the general population as well as samples of infected and high-risk populations; sexual networks we have focused on include both local and partial networks; and our methodologies include both quantitative and qualitative approaches. Our studies focus on three general topics:

1. Description of prevalent sexual mixing patterns, sexual networks, and sexual part-nership types in both quantitative and qualitative terms. The descriptive focus includes attention to methodological issues of data collection and measurement (both quantitative and qualitative), and analysis.
2. Exploration of factors which influence prevalent sexual mixing patterns, sexual networks, and sexual partnership types including (*a*) determinants (both at the level of individual characteristics and partnership characteristics) of observed patterns; (*b*) individual motivations for particular partnership types and mixing patterns; and (*c*) population level demographic, social, and economic factors which influence patterns of sexual mixing, sexual networks, and sexual partner-ship types.
3. Investigation of consequences of patterns of sexual mixing, sexual networks, and sexual partnership types for (*a*) classical STD epidemiology, including the calcula-tion of relative risk for specific STD associated with particular patterns of sexual mixing, sexual networks, and partnership types; determination of population prevalence of particular sexual mixing patterns, sexual networks, sexual partner-ship types and STD, and based on these, the determination of the attributable risk and disease burden associated with specific mixing and network patterns and partnership types; (*b*) STD transmission dynamics, and more specifically, the probability of exposure between infected and uninfected individuals as it is affected by sexual mixing patterns, networks, partnership types, and the duration of infection and the probability of transmission in distinct population subgroups; and (*c*) STD prevention including implications of sexual mixing, sexual networks, and sexual partnership types for STD risk assessment, STD partner notification, and social and behavioral interventions for STD.

The following three data sets are referred to throughout this manuscript.

6.3.1 *Stage I: Clinic-based surveys*

Subjects for Stage I were recruited from two sources. The first source consisted of subjects enrolled in the clinical research core of the UW STD Collaborative Research Center (STDCRC). These were 15–44 year-old English speaking, nonpregnant heterosexual individuals randomly recruited from those seeking care at two STD clinics and one adolescent medicine clinic. From February 1, 1992 to June 1993 all individuals seeking care and meeting the above criteria were eligible. From June 1993 through September 1994 (end of recruitment), the enrollment criteria were narrowed to include only individuals with STD symptoms or history of exposure to an infected partner. A total of 580 individuals with at least one sexual partner within the last 3 months were recruited through the STDCRC.

The second source of subjects for Stage I consisted of individuals with culture confirmed gonococcal or chlamydial infections randomly selected from samples sent to local Nisseria and chlamydia testing labs, respectively. These individuals may have been seen at private or public health facilities. A total of 423 such individuals were recruited. As patients with STD referred their partners for diagnosis and treatment, these individuals were also involved in the study as partners.

Data were collected through standardized face-to-face interviews with respondents and included respondents' demographic and sexual partnership characteristics, their sexual behavior, and the characteristics of their sex partners (as reported by the respondent). In addition, detailed medical history and physical exam data were obtained from the subjects from source 1 (the STDCRC clinical core). Thus, all data included in Stage I lend themselves to local network analyses; and some data on enrolled sex partners lend themselves to partial network analyses.

6.3.2 Stage II: Qualitative data

From June 1996 through June 1998 we interviewed a total of 270 individuals, 150 of which were STD patients with gonorrhea, chlamydial infection, or nongonococcal urethritis and 120 of whom were sampled from the community. Subjects with STD were recruited at the Seattle-King County Department of Public Health STD Clinic at Harborview Medical Center and from private providers in Seattle. A disease intervention specialist (DIS) described the study to eligible individuals after completing the standard partner notification interview. Identifying information for individuals who expressed interest in participation in the study was then provided to study interviewers who arranged for face-to-face interviews. Most of the interviews with patients with STD were conducted within 1 week of the referral from the DIS (69 percent of the men and 73 percent of the women) and only a few were interviewed more than two weeks following the DIS interview (8 percent of men and 15 percent of the women).

In addition to the STD sample, a community sample containing 120 adults 18–50 years of age (of which half were male and the other half female) from six census tracts in metropolitan Seattle, (three with the highest gonorrhea incidence, three randomly selected) was also selected. Twenty individuals were interviewed in each of the six census tracts. Individuals were recruited at grocery stores located in or near each selected census tract because such stores represent a public place utilized by individuals of all demographic and socioeconomic characteristics. Recruitment occurred at different times of the day, and was voluntary. Interview dates and contact information were obtained for individuals who expressed interest at the grocery store and the interviews occurred at the study office. Thus, the interviews that constitute Stage II were based on a quota sample and collected the qualitative data on sexual behavior and sexual partners described later in this paper.

6.3.3 Stage III: Telephone surveys

In Stage III two samples were selected: a random digit dialing (RDD) sample of all Seattle residents aged 18–39 years, and a sample of African-Americans (AA) from individuals with listed telephone numbers ("listed sample"). There probably was a loss of poorer individuals but we did not measure this. An additional sample of AA was selected because they have higher rates of STD both nationally and in Seattle, and national data suggest that STD morbidity and sexual practices differ between AA and White Americans (WA). A total of 356 WA and 140 AA individuals who had ever engaged in vaginal intercourse answered questions regarding their demographics, sexual behavior, sexual history, STD history, and most recent heterosexual partner. Interviews averaged 21 min in length. The cooperation rate was 67.5 percent for the RDD sample and 28.2 percent for the AA sample, which was considerably lower than we had hoped for. Questions on partners' characteristics were formulated to elicit information on the most recent four partners. Specific sex partner parameters included date of first and last sex, partner's age, race-ethnicity, employment status, and education.

6.3.4 Sampling concerns

Only a few studies of sexual mixing and sexual partnership characteristics have been based on population-based samples (Laumann et al. 1994; Foxman and Holmes 1995). Instead, most studies utilize convenience samples or random samples from some subpopulation (i.e. individuals attending an STD clinic). There are advantages and disadvantages of each approach, depending on the primary scientific questions of interest. Population-based samples give unbiased estimates of mixing parameters and are important if one is developing a mixing-dependent model of disease spread for some population. However, it would require an inordinately large sample size to get enough STD's in a population-based sample to draw conclusions about mixing and risk of STD.

In addition, in the United States, mixing in the general population is largely irrelevant to the spread of many STDs which are confined to core groups. Thus, studies in at-risk populations are necessary to understand the relationship between mixing and the persistence and spread of many STDs. A key question, then, is how to relate such samples to the general population? One approach might be to view samples from STD clinics and other high-risk populations as an oversample of a particular subgroup of the main population. By combining information from various sources it might be possible, with appropriate weighting, to reconstruct estimates of mixing and its relationship to STD that are both unbiased and precise. Further research into such an approach is required, however.

6.4 FIELDWORK EXPERIENCES

Interviewers were disease intervention specialists (Stage I), graduate students (Stage II), and professional interviewers (Stage III) all of whom were specifically trained to administer the specific data collection instruments used in our studies.

6.4.1 Eligibility criteria for STD patients

More than half of the sample for our second stage studies is composed of STD patients. The eligibility criteria specified men and women with gonorrhea or chlamydial infection, or men with nongonoccocal urethritis. The challenge of recruiting such individuals to a study is that individuals presenting with symptoms typical of exposure to gonorrhea or chlamydia are often treated presumptively when they seek care, before a laboratory diagnosis; or they may be tested for gonorrhea and chlamydia at the time of the visit and once the laboratory results become available the appropriate medication is called in to a pharmacy for the patient to pick up at his/her convenience. In either scenario, patients are advised to return to the clinic to be retested in a few weeks, but many do not reappear. Therefore, during the study recruitment period, a definitive diagnosis of gonorrhea and chlamydia often could not be made at the time patients sought care at the clinic. Once the laboratory results became available, patients who did not return to the clinic for follow up were called by telephone and informed of their results. Thus, many patients were recruited for the study *after* their initial visit—not at the time that they were experiencing STD symptoms or were concerned about exposure and seeking testing. Some patients could never be recontacted and others were simply not interested in returning to a place near the clinic or even the clinic itself for the study at a later date. We may have lost many potential subjects due to having to wait for laboratory results before recruiting patients.

The eligibility criteria caused a second problem in recruitment—the actual "recruiters" for the study were the individuals who informed STD patients of their laboratory results and recontacted patients after their initial visit for this purpose. These were the DISs who also are responsible for conducting partner notification interviews at the time of providing STD results. It is possible that the interview concerning partner notification may be perceived as more contentious than our interviews concerning partnerships for patients not willing to disclose partners, that is, identities for partner notification. Therefore, the personnel who conducted the recruitment may have served as a further barrier to study enrollment.

The final problem was that recruitment was a multiphased process; DIS first had to ascertain potential subjects eligibility, and then gain their permission to be contacted for the study. Next a study interviewer had to recontact the individual (often a challenge) and set up an appointment for an interview. A considerable number of subjects never appeared for the scheduled interview.

6.4.2 Identification of "main partner" in interview

The qualitative interview delved deeply into subject's sexual partnership histories and collected detailed information on the current or most recent main partner as well as other important partnerships. For some subjects, identification of one partner or another as main was not possible. When directly asked if the subject currently had a main partner, a complicated description of a series of current partners often unfolded. Such descriptions often became convoluted and confusing so that the interviewer might have decided for the respondent who to call the main partner and then proceed with the next segment of the interview on the main partnership dynamics for that partner. During the coding of the interview it was often a challenge to mark one such partnership as main, and yet coding more than one as main became too confusing for the analysis. In some interviews, a subject would provide detailed and extremely descriptive information about one partnership, and then later in the interview start referring to another partner who was clearly also current and important. The interviewer and later the coder often became confused as to whether to return to the same questions about the main partnership and how to identify this second (or third) partner. The same problem arose with both male and female subjects. This problem arose more often in interviews with STD patients but often occurred in the interviews from the community (general population) although usually with young respondents, 18–25 years of age. This confusion may have resulted from our a priori assumption that partners could be clearly classified as main and non-main partners.

6.4.3 *Over reporting and exaggeration*

Qualitative interviews were all conducted by gender-matched interviewers. The same two interviewers conducted all 270 interviews throughout the study and were both social work graduate students with experience of working with high-risk populations. Nevertheless, there may have been dynamics created within the interviews resulting in subjects feeling a need to over report numbers of sex partners or their practice of safe sex behavior. For example, some subjects claimed to have had all potential sex partners tested for STDs before engaging in sexual activity with them. However, given the time between meeting such partners and first sex, a visit to the STD clinic and obtaining laboratory test results was not feasible. Additionally, some male subjects may have been influenced by a desire to impress the male interviewer with their own virility. This possible interviewer bias must be balanced, however, against the excellent rapport that this interviewer established with most subjects and his ability to engage subjects in great self-disclosure. While most female subjects seemed experienced and comfortable in engaging in detailed discussions of their sexual partnerships, this was not an experience that many males expressed.

6.4.4 *Transcription burden*

The final challenge of qualitative data collection was the burden of transcribing these extremely detailed and long qualitative interviews into verbatim text. Each interview was a minimum of a half an hour in duration and the average length was 45 minutes. Most interviews took about 3 h to transcribe. Hiring professional transcribers proved not only too expensive, but also created extra work as most had difficulty understanding the respondents and often summarized rather than transcribed verbatim, requiring complete review and revision of all transcribed interviews.

Therefore, the interviewers were assigned responsibility for transcribing their own interviews, which resulted in more accurate transcriptions but not in the most efficient manner.

6.5 METHODOLOGICAL ISSUES

6.5.1 Analyses based on mixing matrices

Mixing matrices are commonly used to summarize patterns of sexual mixing. A mixing matrix is a cross tabulation of a characteristic (e.g. race) of a respondent (or index case) with the corresponding characteristic of the partner (Fig. 6.2).

Mixing matrices are used to evaluate the *degree* of assortative (like-with-like) versus disassortative (like-with-unlike) mixing and for determining *patterns* of disassortative mixing. One may envision a variety of possible measures of the degree of assortativeness. The proportion of individuals falling on the main diagonal of the mixing matrix is known as the concordance or homophily rate. Formally,

$$C = \sum_i p_{ii}$$

where C is concordance and $p_{ij} = n_{ij}/N$. If each respondent contributes only one partner to the mixing matrix, then var(C) is given by

$$\mathrm{var}(C) = \left(\sum_i p_{ii}(1 - p_{ii}) - \sum_{ij} p_{ii}p_{jj} \right) \Big/ N$$

If each respondent contributes multiple partners, then the estimate of the variance must account for the potential dependence between the multiple partners of each respondent. The concordance varies from 0 to 1 and has a simple probabilistic interpretation: it is the probability that a randomly chosen respondent–partner pair is concordant with respect to the characteristic of interest.

A disadvantage of C as a measure of assortativeness is that it does not differentiate between assortativeness due to intentional partner selection versus assortativeness due to chance alone (random mixing). For instance, in a racially homogeneous population one would expect high concordance even if respondents were not consciously selecting partners according to their race. Thus, variations in concordance may be due to variations in partner availability rather than variations in partner selection.

Partner characteristic category

		1	2	...	I	Total
Respondent	1	n_{11}	n_{12}	...	n_{1I}	$n_{1.}$
Characteristic	:	:	:		:	:
Category	I	n_{I1}	n_{I2}	...	n_{II}	$n_{I.}$
Total		$n_{.1}$	$n_{.2}$	...	$n_{.I}$	N

Figure 6.2. *Mixing Matrix*

In epidemiology a common chance-corrected measure of agreement (assortative-ness) is the kappa statistic. In this context, the kappa statistic may be written as

$$\kappa = \frac{\sum_i p_{i.}(p_{i|i} - p_{.i})}{\sum_i p_{i.}(1 - p_{.i})} \tag{1}$$

where $p_{i.}$ is the marginal probability that the respondent characteristic is in category i ($Pr(res = i) = n_{i.}/N$), $p_{.i}$ is the marginal probability that the partner characteristic is in category i ($Pr(ptr = i) = n_{.i}/N$) and $p_{j|i}$ is the conditional probability that the partner is in category j given that the respondent is in category i ($Pr(ptr = j|res = i) = n_{ij}/n_{.i}$). Note that C may be viewed as a special case of kappa in which the chance-corrections have been removed (i.e. setting all $p_{.i} = 0$ in eqn (1) gives C since $p_{ii} = p_{i|i}p_{i.}$).

A disadvantage of using kappa in the study of mixing matrices is that, unless the sample represents a probability sample from the general population, the marginal probability distributions of the respondent and the partner characteristic in the sample ($p_{i.}$ and $p_{.i}$, respectively) will usually not reflect the distribution of those characteristics in the population. Thus, the chance-corrections ($p_{.i}$) in eqn (1) do not reflect the true partner availability rates. If knowledge of the population distribution of the characteristic of interest is available from other sources, then it may be possible to use this information in eqn (1) to derive a chance corrected measure of assortativeness. An alternative approach to this problem was taken by Gupta and Anderson (1989) and others in their studies of mixing matrices. They define a chance-corrected measure of assortativeness known as Q:

$$Q = \frac{\sum_i p_{i|i} - 1}{I - 1}$$

where I is the number of categories in the mixing matrix. It is straightforward to show that Q is a special case of kappa in which $p_{i.} = 1/I$ for all categories i. In addition, when $p_{i.} = 1/I$ for all i, the marginal distribution of the partner characteristics, $p_{.i}$ is irrelevant (see eqn (1)). Thus, Q avoids the problem of estimating the population distributions of the respondent and partner characteristics by standardizing to a particular (uniform) distribution of the respondent characteristic. Q varies from a minimum of $-1/(I-1)$ to 1.0. Random partner selection (random mixing) gives $Q = 0$ (the reverse is not necessarily true, however). Assortative mixing gives values of Q greater than 0 while disassortative mixing gives values less than 0.

Since the rows of the mixing matrix represent independent samples, the variance of Q may be readily derived. If each respondent contributes only one partnership to the mixing matrix, then we have

$$\begin{aligned} \text{var}(Q) &= \frac{\sum_i \text{var}(p_{i|i})}{(I-1)^2} \\ &= \frac{\sum_i p_{i|i}(1 - p_{i|i})/n_{i.}}{(I-1)^2}. \end{aligned} \tag{2}$$

If respondents contribute multiple partnerships to the mixing matrix then the variance of the p_{ili} must be adjusted for correlated data (e.g. using generalized estimating equations, Liang and Zeger 1986).

The above measures summarize the mixing matrix as a whole with respect to assortativeness. However, they give little information on the patterns of assortativeness or disassortativeness. Morris (1991) uses log-linear modeling methods to examine various hypotheses regarding patterns of mixing. In particular, she defines the following hierarchy of models for mixing: (*a*) proportional (random) mixing; (*b*) uniform homophily in which respondents preferentially select partners similar to themselves but select dissimilar partners at random; the in-group preference is identical for all respondents; (*c*) differential homophily in which respondents preferentially select partners similar to themselves but select dissimilar partners at random; the in-group preference is different for each respondent group; and (*d*) arbitrary selection pattern (Morris 1991). In preliminary analyses of our racial mixing data, we find strong support for the differential homophily model.

Mixing matrices are natural summaries of assortativeness for measures which are discrete in nature such as race, religion, and, perhaps, educational attainment. However, for measures that are continuous in nature such as age and number of sex partners over long periods, categorization into discrete intervals can result in arbitrary variations in measures of assortativeness. As a general rule, dividing a continuous variable into more categories will reduce estimates of assortativeness. Predicting the effect of varying the choice of cutpoints is more difficult, however. In addition, categorizing a continuous measure can lead to apparent anomalies such as calling a 19-year-old respondent with a 20-year-old partner "discordant" while a 25-year-old respondent with a 20-year-old partner might be labeled concordant. One solution to this problem is to simply classify partnerships into two categories—concordant or discordant—depending on the degree of difference (absolute or relative) between the respondent and his or her partner for the characteristic of interest. An extension to this idea is to classify the partnership into three categories—concordant, discordant low, and discordant high—depending on the direction of the discordance.

An alternative, and perhaps more natural, measure of concordance for continuous measures is the concordance correlation coefficient (Lin 1989), which avoids arbitrary divisions into categories. The concordance correlation is defined as

$$\rho_c = \frac{2\sigma_{12}}{\sigma_1^2 + \sigma_2^2 + (\mu_1 - \mu_2)^2}$$

where $\sigma_{12}, \sigma_1^2, \sigma_2^2, \mu_1,$ and μ_2 are the covariance, the variances and the means of the respondents and the partners, respectively. The concordance correlation measures the spread around a 45° line in a scatterplot of the respondent characteristic versus the partner characteristic. If the points in the scatterplot fall close to the 45° line, then the concordance correlation will be close to 1.0. If the points do not fall close to the 45° line, then the concordance correlation will be small. If the population means and variances are identical (and since the labeling of one member of the partnership as respondent and one as partner is arbitrary this seems reasonable for characteristics like age) then this measure is equal to the usual Pearson correlation coefficient. It can also be shown that for discrete measures (e.g. race) the concordance correlation reduces to the kappa statistic.

In studies of sexual mixing, it is natural to want to relate mixing patterns to risk of STDs. One approach is presented in Aral et al. (1999, table 4), in which the relative risk of STD is computed for respondents in discordant partnerships relative to respondents in concordant partnerships. Separate relative risks were computed for race, age, education and number of previous partners and, within, each dimension, for male and female respondents. The analytic tool for these analyses was generalized estimating equations (GEE), an extension of logistic regression for correlated data. Adjustment of the estimated relative risks for confounders and/or effect modifiers is theoretically possible by including these in the regression model, but lack of sufficient data will generally constrain these efforts.

6.5.2 Estimating partnership "duration"

Characterizing partnerships and partnership duration is important for two reasons. First, the current duration of a partnership (the length of time since the individuals began having sex, also referred to below as *recency*) may influence the risk of STD. If recency is a risk factor for STD then it may be of interest to estimate and compare the distribution of current partnership durations in some population or subpopulations. Second, deterministic mathematical models of disease spread typically treat sexual partnerships as "instantaneous" entities and ignore the issue of sexual partnership duration. A good mathematical characterization of sexual partnerships could lead to improved epidemic models. In this case, we wish to characterize the total partnership duration as opposed to the current partnership duration. In the following we describe the data we have available for these purposes and the analytic challenges in estimating both recency and total partnership duration.

Participants in the Stage I studies were asked to describe each partner with whom they had sex in the last 3 months. Information available on each partner includes the date the partner and respondent first had sex, the date of last sex, and the estimated number of sex acts over that time period. Although these data can be used to estimate recency of partnership formation (i.e. current duration), total duration, and sexual activity levels over the course of a partnership, naïve estimates of these quantities will be severely biased. To understand this, consider Fig. 6.3 and the problem of estimating current partnership duration. When only active partnerships are assessed there is a bias towards including partnerships of longer duration. That is, among all partnerships that began at some fixed time point—say, 12 months prior to assessment—only those that are still active (the longest lasting ones) will be included in the sample. This process is known as left truncation (because it truncates the left-hand tail of the distribution of partnership durations, which corresponds to shorter partnerships) and it biases estimates of current duration upwards. In the statistical literature, this is known as "delayed entry" and is an example of length-biased sampling. In the AIDS/HIV literature the term "prevalent cohort bias" is used to describe a similar problem.

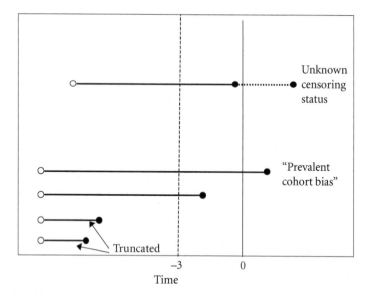

Figure 6.3. *Collection of Partnership Duration and Frequency Data*

It is possible to develop estimates that correct for this bias. Suppose Y_i is the observed (current) duration of the ith partnership (i.e. the time from the start of the partnership to the date of last sex). The corrected product limit (Kaplan–Meier) estimator of the survival distribution of current duration at time t is given by

$$Pr(\text{Duration} > t) = S(t) = \prod_{Y_i \leq t}\left(1 - \frac{1}{R(Y_i)}\right)$$

where $R(y) = \Sigma_i I(l_i \leq y) - I(Y_i < y)$ and l_i is the truncation time of the ith partnership (i.e. the time from the start of the partnership to the beginning of the observation period). $I(x)$ is the indicator function with value 1 if x is true and 0 otherwise. Effectively, $R(Y_i)$ counts the number of individuals at risk of failure at the time that subject i failed, thus, $1/R(Y_i)$ is the proportion of individuals failing at time Y_i and $1 - 1/R(Y_i)$ is the proportion of individuals surviving. Some statistical packages (e.g. SPLUS and SAS) can compute this estimator of the survival function using the "counting process" method of representing survival time data.

Similar problems are encountered when trying to estimate the distribution of total duration or the evolution of sexual frequency over the course of a partnership (in the latter case, the partnerships with zero frequency are truncated by the observation scheme). An additional issue when trying to estimate total duration is that a "censoring" indicator is required to determine if the partnership is still active at the time of the visit. In studies of partnership duration, it is useful to ask "Is this partnership ongoing?" (although such a measure of censoring would probably be subject to some degree of error). In our studies this question was not asked so only respondents who returned for follow-up visits and gave information about their partnerships at that time provide information about total duration.

Assuming that partnerships form and dissolve according to some duration distribution (i.e. the distribution of total duration discussed above) leads to a simple abstract description of a sexual partnership but tells us nothing about the frequency of sexual activity within the partnership, which may be important in models of disease transmission. In addition, the concept of duration in general presupposes that sexual partnerships have a well-defined endpoint, which is often not the case. An alternative approach to characterizing sexual partnerships is by using the concept of sexual frequency. Sexual frequency is defined as the rate of sex acts per unit time. From this point of view, partnerships do not explicitly end; rather, the frequency drops to zero for an indefinite period. The available data provide a collection of 3-month windows of observations on sexual frequency at random points after the start of the partnership. From cross-sectional data of this sort (i.e. one 3-month retrospective observation period per partnership) one can reconstruct the population average frequency across all partnerships over time. A limitation, however, is that all the frequency data are conditional on the current frequency being greater than zero (the zero-truncation problem alluded to above).

In other words, partnerships are only included in the sample if the sexual frequency at the time of sampling is greater than zero. While the frequency of sexual contacts among active partnerships is of interest in its own right, one would also like to estimate the proportion of partnerships, which are currently active (i.e. frequency greater than zero). There are two solutions to this problem. One possibility is to use only partnerships that formed during the initial 3-month window of observation or during follow-up. There is no loss of data due to truncation in these partnerships. Figure 6.4 shows the results of such an analysis from the existing sex partner networks data set. However, this analysis uses only a fraction of the available data and can only follow partnerships out to a maximum of the length of follow-up plus the length of the pre-enrollment window (e.g. in the sex partner networks study this is 15 months—12 months of follow-up plus 3 months prior to the entry visit). To make full use of the data we propose developing self-consistent estimators (Turnbull 1976) which will adjust for the zero-truncation bias described above. This approach to estimation is closely related to the estimate of the duration distribution with left truncation given above.

Frequency curves that have been estimated in the manner described above can be compared across subgroups. Comparisons between subgroups of partnerships that are defined by an attribute that does not vary over time can be compared using a permutation test. One would first define a measure of the difference between two curves (e.g. mean absolute distance between the curves or maximum difference). The observed value of this difference measure would be compared to the distribution of differences obtained when the attribute of interest is randomly permuted among the partnerships. If the observed difference has low probability under the permutation

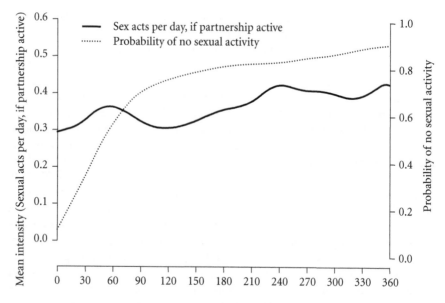

Figure 6.4. *Sexual Frequency Over Time*

distribution then this is evidence against the null hypothesis of no difference between the subgroups.

The curves shown in Fig. 6.4 represent the mean sexual frequency across the population. To model the temporal evolution of sexual frequency on the individual partnership level will require longitudinal data.

6.6 KEY FINDINGS

Over the past decade our team has analyzed various Seattle data sets in search of answers to many questions including:

1. What are the mixing patterns of STD clinic attendees with respect to age, race-ethnicity, education, number of sex partners?
2. What are the mixing patterns of the Seattle general population?
3. Are the sexual partnership characteristics of individuals infected with STD similar to or different from the sexual partnership characteristics of individuals who do not have STD?
4. Do sex partner risk profiles accurately reflect partners' behaviors (to what extent can we depend on ego-centered data on partners characteristics and behaviors)?
5. Is mixing with other racial ethnic groups associated with increased or decreased relative risk of being diagnosed with gonorrhea? chlamydial infection? genital warts? genital herpes?

6. Is mixing with other age groups associated with increased or decreased relative risk of being diagnosed with specific sexually transmitted infections (STIs)?
7. Are the sexual networks of individuals infected with gonorrhea similar to or different from the sexual networks of individuals infected with chlamydia?
8. What are the similarities and differences between the ways in which mixing patterns influence relative risk of bacterial *versus* viral STDs? Curable *versus* not-curable STDs?
9. Based on qualitative data, what are some of the motives that lead individuals into specific types of sexual partnerships and/or sexual networks (those associated with high or low risk for acquisition of STIs)

Some of these analyses have employed quantitative data analyses while others have focused on data collected through in-depth interviews using qualitative approaches. Some of our findings on the descriptives, determinants, motivations, and consequences of sexual networks are summarized below.

6.6.1 *Quantitative descriptive findings*

To describe variations in sociodemographic and behavioral sex partner concordance (SPC) by demographic characteristics, sexual behavior, infection status, and partnership characteristics in our study population of STD clinic attendees, we analyzed SPC data using GEE, logistic regression and GEE linear regression (Aral et al. 1995). Five hundred and eighty randomly selected patients seeking care in three Seattle clinics reported on a total of 1286 unique respondent–partner dyads over a follow-up period of up to 1 year during face-to-face interviews.

The highest level of SPC was observed with respect to age (0.78) and the lowest with respect to number of partners (0.60). SPC with respect to race/ethnicity (0.74) and education (0.71) lay in between. Multivariate analyses revealed complex interactions among behavioral and demographic characteristics and SPC. Persons with a history of laboratory evidence of STIs were least likely to have sex partners of their own race/ethnicity and least likely to be concordant with partners for lifetime number of sex partners.

Preliminary comparisons of sexual mixing patterns of Seattle STD clinic attendees with patterns of the general population of Seattle suggested that high-risk populations engage in relationships less concordant with respect to race/ethnicity, age, number of partners and social class parameters such as education and income (Aral et al. 1995). A telephone survey was conducted on a random digit dialed (RDD) sample of the Seattle population, and an AA over sample selected from census tracks with 40 percent or more AA households (Stage III) (Foxman and Holmes 1995). The kappa statistic was used to examine the agreement between respondents and their most recent sex partner with respect to age, race, education, and lifetime number of sex partners. The highest kappa observed (0.36) was for agreement in age and the lowest level (0.15) was for agreement in lifetime number of sex partners. Kappa values for agreement in race/ethnicity (0.21) and education (0.25) were in the middle.

A comparison of these data to the national data reported by Laumann et al. (1994) suggests variations in mixing patterns across local areas and differences between national findings and local findings (Aral et al. 1995). For example, levels of race/ ethnicity concordance between sex partners were consistently higher for the national sample than they were for the Seattle general population sample. These differences were particularly marked for AA men and women, and Asian men and women, indicating greater mixing across race/ethnicity boundaries for the Seattle general population. Unlike those in the national sample, AA women in Seattle did not have the highest concordance in race/ethnicity in their partnerships; and the gender differential between white men and women seen in the NHSLS did not exist in Seattle—white men and women were equally likely to be in partnerships with other whites. These findings suggest relatively more open sexual mixing patterns in Seattle compared to the national population.

In one analysis of Stage I data we tried to determine if SPC with respect to race/ ethnicity, age, education, and number of partners among sex partnerships with a history of chlamydial infection is different from SPC with respect to race/ethnicity, age, education, and number of partners among sex partnerships with a history of infection with gonorrhea and syphilis, and sex partnerships with no history of infection (Aral et al. 1994). We analyzed data collected in face-to-face interviews with 461 patients seeking care in Seattle clinics. They reported a total of 979 unique respondent–partner dyads. We found greater SPC for patients with a history of chlamydial infection than for patients with a history of gonorrhea or syphilis. Persons with a history of chlamydia were most likely, and persons with a history of gonorrhea or syphilis were least likely to have sex with others similar to themselves with respect to race/ ethnicity, age, and education. Persons with a history of any one of the three infections were less likely than people with no history of infection to have sex with people similar to themselves with respect to number of lifetime partners. These findings suggest that people with a history of chlamydia infection, like people with no history of chlamydia, gonorrhea, or syphilis, tend to choose sex partners of the same race/ ethnicity as themselves, while people with a history of gonorrhea or syphilis are less likely to do so. People with a history of chlamydial infection are also more likely to choose partners similar to themselves in age and education compared to those with gonorrhea and syphilis, but these differences seemed due to differences in the age, sex, and education of the respondents in these subgroups. People with a history of chlamydial infection, and those with a history of gonorrhea or syphilis, compared to those with no history of chlamydia, gonorrhea, or syphilis were more likely to have sex partners *unlike* themselves with respect to number of lifetime partners.

Brunham and Plummer (1990) have estimated, based on information available about the mean durations of infectivity and efficiencies of transmission of various STIs, that the mean rate of partner change is highest for individuals with syphilis, intermediate for those with gonorrhea and chlamydia, and lowest for genital herpes (Brunham and Plummer 1990). We attempted to determine networks of sexual activity and rates of sex partner change for heterosexual patients with syphilis, gonorrhea, chlamydia, and genital herpes infections in King County (Stoner et al. 1993). Based on contact tracing information obtained in Stage I data set, networks were defined as clusters of infected index cases and their named sexual contacts. Our results were consistent with earlier estimates: individuals within syphilis networks reported the highest mean number of sexual contacts in the previous 90-day period (4.0), followed by persons within gonorrhea (2.9), chlamydia (1.8), and herpes (1.0) networks. Greater numbers of partners within the previous 90 days were reported by men (mean 3.1, median 2.0) than by women (mean 2.3, median 1.5) ($p < .01$). These findings support the hypothesis that syphilis and gonorrhea require higher rates of partner change to sustain the spread of infection than do chlamydia and herpes infection.

We also evaluated sociodemographic and behavioral factors, which correlated with membership in networks of gonococcal and chlamydial transmission, using contact tracing information collected in the Stage I data set (Stoner et al. 2000). Data from face-to-face interviews with 127 gonorrhea patients and 184 chlamydia patients (index cases) and their named sex partners, as well as the partners of infected partners were analyzed. Gonococcal network members differed significantly from chlamydial network members in a number of demographic variables, including race/ethnicity, education, and unemployment status. Gonococcal network members were more likely to report prior history of crack–cocaine use, sexual assault, and having been in jail. Gonococcal network members also reported more sex partners in the past 1 year and past 3 months than did chlamydial network members. Gonococcal and chlamydial mixing matrices demonstrated assortativeness for sex partner selection by race/ethnicity but not by sexual activity level, and no systematic differences between networks were noted. Gonococcal networks were larger than chlamydial networks.

Accurate assessment of sex partner risk behaviors is important for minimizing STD/HIV risk to self as well as to future partners. Few data are available to address whether a respondent's perceptions of sex partner risk profiles accurately reflect partners' behaviors. We compared STD patients' risk assessments of partners with partners' behaviors as reported by partners (Stoner et al. 1997). Detailed face-to-face interviews with 151 index cases with gonorrhea or chlamydial infection and their named sex partners in Seattle yielded 191 unique relationship dyads. Index cases were queried about perceived sex partner sociodemographic and behavioral characteristics, and perceptions were then sociometrically validated by direct comparison with partner self-reports.

Of 115 partners perceived to be monogamous in the past 3 months, 42 (35.3 percent) reported having two or more partners during the same time frame. This effect was independent of gender, age, race/ethnicity, or duration of presexual relationship. Perceptions of partners' lifetime numbers of partners correlated poorly with partner self-reports ($r^2 = 0.06$), and nearly half (48.6 percent) of all index cases underestimated the actual number stated by partners by 25 percent or more. Of 152 partners, 6 partners (3.9 percent) acknowledged having sex with prostitutes and of 170 partners, 6 partners (3.5 percent) admitted past or current IV drug use, although these behaviors were not perceived by index cases. Potentially protective characteristics were also misperceived: 14 or 93 male partners (15.1 percent) thought to be circumcised by index cases were uncircumcised. We conclude that STD patients' perceptions of sex partner risk behaviors were not often highly consistent with self-reports of partners with whom they were not involved in established, ongoing relationships.

6.6.2 *Qualitative descriptive findings*

Social processes underlying sex partner selection and partnership formation—basic social processes that lead to the formation of sex partnership networks—are poorly understood. In order to better describe (and understand) these processes, we have been examining the social context of partnership formation, maintenance, and dissolution (Gorbach et al. 1997). Thus far, we have analyzed data from in-depth, semistructured interviews conducted with 150 persons with gonorrhea and chlamydia (STD sample) and 120 persons from a community sample (270 total) included in the Stage II data set. Interviews explored respondent's context of sex partner selection and recruitment, and were loosely structured to allow for probing and follow-up questioning of respondents by a gender-matched interviewer. All interviews were tape-recorded and transcribed verbatim, and a formal content analysis performed to identify recurrent themes.

The following themes were identified in a preliminary analysis of twenty persons with gonorrhea or with chlamydial infection (STD sample) and twenty persons from the community sample:

1. Community sample respondents tended to be monogamous and most reported having a primary sex partner. By contrast, in the STD sample greater diversity of sexual partnerships and fewer primary partners were reported;
2. Respondents in both samples reported a myriad of sexual partnership types, including long term casual, "bootycall", and sex-for-drugs with "strawberries";
3. STD respondents found partners outside their social networks more often than those from the community sample;
4. Concurrent partnerships were more common and more recent in the STD than in the community sample. Factors associated with concurrent partnerships were partners' incarceration, illicit drug use, and reappearance of past partners. These findings suggest greater disparity between social and sexual networks and more frequent partnership concurrency for persons with gonorrhea or with chlamydial infection.

6.6.3 *Determinants*

Concurrent partnerships fuel the spread of STIs in populations (Morris and Kretzschmar 1997). There is no evidence in the literature regarding the determinants of partnership concurrency. To explore factors which may influence concurrency, we analyzed data from the random digit-dial telephone survey ($n = 544$ responses) on sexual behavior of Seattle residents aged 18–39 years; the Stage III data set (Manhart et al. 2002). A further sample of AA respondents was added ($n = 144$), to provide sufficient numbers to explore reported differences in STD rates and sexual behavior (see Foxman et al. 1998, for a description of sampling procedures). The analysis was restricted to sexually active individuals whose most recent sexual partnership was heterosexual. We studied both individual characteristics that are associated with individuals' likelihood of having concurrent partnerships; and partnership characteristics associated with either partner reporting concurrent partnerships.

To assess prevalence of and compare different methods of defining concurrency we collected four types of information. Respondents were asked about (*a*) start and end dates of their most recent and next-to-last sexual relationships (to calculate overlap); (*b*) the length of time between sexual partners in days, weeks, months, or years (gap); (*c*) the number of people with whom they had sexual contact while they were involved in a sexual partnership with their most recent partner (multiple concurrent partners); and (*d*) whether the respondent believed his/her partner had other partners during the sexual relationship.

When asked directly if they had any other partners during their sexual relationship with their most recent partner (multiple concurrent partners), more men than women responded affirmatively (26.7 versus 17.7 percent). Slightly more women than men believed that their partners had other partners (17.6 versus 15.1 percent). However, when partnership concurrency was defined as the belief partner was unfaithful or respondent had multiple concurrent partners, slightly more men than women were classified as being in a concurrent partnership (27.0 and 24.0 percent, respectively). Combining information on overlap, multiple concurrent partners, and belief the partner had, other partners categorized the highest proportion of individuals as concurrent (38.7 percent of male respondents and 32.4 percent of female respondents), while combining information on gap between partners, multiple concurrent partners, and belief the partner had, others classified slightly lower proportions of both men (33.1 percent) and women (27.1 percent) as concurrent. Although the combinations including the overlap information and the gap information increased the proportion of concurrent partnerships, this effect may have been partially due to misclassification of individuals as concurrent who actually had short gaps between partnerships.

For both men and women, having ever had a same sex partner, having ever spent a night in jail, increasing lifetime number of sex partners, and engaging in a wider variety of sexual practices were individual characteristics associated with having concurrent sex partners. In addition, among men, being divorced, widowed, or separated, being unemployed; and having a history of self-reported STD prior to the most recent partnership; and among women, being unemployed, reporting young age at sexual debut, and self-reported diagnosis of STD in the most recent partnership were associated with having concurrent sex partners. Individuals' age, income, education, or race/ethnicity were not associated with concurrency. Partnership characteristics that were associated with concurrent partnerships included higher partnership order, either partner having spent a night in jail, and time elapsed between meeting and engaging in sexual intercourse. Being married and living together were associated with lower proportion of concurrency. Partnerships marked by age or educational differences were not more likely to be concurrent.

6.6.4 Individual motivations

In order to understand the nature of partnerships patients with STD participated in, it is important to describe the meanings different partnership types have for them and the functions they perform. To understand motivations associated with concurrency, we analyzed Stage II data from in-depth, semistructured interviews conducted with 150 persons with gonorrhea, chlamydia, or nongonococcal urethritis recruited from an STD clinic, and 120 persons from a community sample of adults over 18 years of age (Gorbach 2000). Our results indicate that in certain social groups there is an expectation that one partner is not enough to fulfill one's social, economic, and personal needs. Concurrency may reflect a strategy of sexual networking undertaken in situations of perceived economic or social shortages in which sexual partnerships are necessary for survival. We interviewed male and female patients with STD, male and female members of high STD risk communities, and male and female members of low STD risk communities. History of concurrent partnerships were reported by all the groups studied. The most common type of concurrent partnership was overlapping short-term partnerships. Other types of concurrent partnerships reported fell into the following categories: physical separation from main partner, transition between partners, reactive nonmonogamy within a partnership, reciprocal nonmonogamy (open partnership), and alternating main partners.

Concurrency was clustered around specific ages including the early twenties and mid-forties. This pattern is apparently inconsistent with our findings based on analyses of Stage III data described earlier. This may result from the focus of Stage II data on current partnership concurrencies while Stage III data reflected the cumulative experience over a longer time period. Men in all groups reported utilizing concurrent partnerships as a strategy to avoid being partnerless at the disintegration of a partnership; women, especially female STD patients, reported more reactive nonmonogamy and sequestering new partners themselves rather than dissolving the partnership when they realize their partners have other partners. No low risk women and only one male STD patient of all the men studied reported the latter pattern. Concurrency that is due to physical separation or that arises during a transition between partners was not perceived as violating norms of monogamy and was reported as a socially acceptable form of nonmonogamy.

Ever and past year concurrent partnerships were reported by 80 and 57 percent of male STD patients, 80 and 62 percent of female STD patients, 80 and 30 percent of high STD risk community men, 63 and 10 percent of low STD risk community men, 63 and 20 percent of high STD risk community women, and 50 and 20 percent of low STD risk community women, respectively.

These findings suggest that in some social groups there is an expectation that one partner is not enough to fulfill one's social, economic, and personal needs. Concurrency may reflect a strategy of sexual networking undertaken in situations of perceived economic or social shortages, where sexual partnerships facilitate survival. Some form of concurrent partnerships were found in all groups studied, suggesting some patterns of concurrency are socially acceptable but are linked to the life stage of individuals. Concurrency in some forms may be more open to public health messages than others (e.g. those in which partners have little control over the dynamics around sexual behavior in their partnerships). STD programs developing intervention messages targeting concurrent partnerships need to recognize that concurrency is a survival mechanism for some and in some settings may be a socially acceptable pattern (Gorbach et al. 2000).

We have also analyzed the qualitative data described above (Stage II) to explore the varied aspects of partner selection and partnership formation processes among men with varying risk for STD, in order to address the issues of content scripting and social exchange aspects of sexual relationships within these contexts (Stoner et al. 2003). Our preliminary findings suggest that formation of sexual partnerships may be associated with STD risk among men; weak social network ties and short presexual periods being correlated with increased STD risk.

6.6.5 Consequences

Patterns of sexual mixing, sexual networks, and sexual partnership types have important consequences for STD relative risk and disease burden for STD, for the modeling of STD transmission dynamics and for STD prevention.

Based on data from Stage I, we sought to define among STD clinic attendees, patterns of sex partner selection, relative risks for gonococcal or chlamydial infection associated with each mixing pattern, and selected links and potential and actual bridge populations (Aral et al. 1998; Aral et al. 1999). Mixing matrices were computed based on characteristics of the study participants and their partners. Risk of infection was determined in study participants with various types of partners, and odds ratios were used to estimate relative risk of infection for discordant versus concordant partnerships. Partnerships discordant in terms of race/ethnicity, age, education, and number of partners were associated with significantly increased risk for gonorrhea and chlamydial infection. In low-prevalence subpopulations, within-subpopulation mixing was associated with chlamydial infection, and direct links with high-prevalence subpopulations were associated with gonorrhea. Our results demonstrate that mixing patterns influence the risk of specific infections, and they should be included in risk assessments for individuals and in the design of screening, health education, and partner notification strategies for populations.

Theoretical studies (Aral et al. 1995) have highlighted the importance of patterns of choice of sex partner in the transmission and persistence of STDs. To describe reported patterns of sexual mixing according to numbers of sex partners and to see how these patterns affect transmission dynamics, we analyzed data from Stage I interviews with patients attending public health clinics in Seattle about their own and their partners' behaviors and sex partner choices (Garnett et al. 1996). Patterns of sexual mixing were weakly assortative. Across activity groups many respondents believed their partners had no other sexual contacts. Those with three or more partners frequently perceived their partners to have three or more partners as well. Persons of high sexual activity who mix assortatively act as a "core group" and make the persistence of STD in a population likely. In addition, because mixing is not highly assortative, a steady trickle of infection from members of the core group will pass to other segments of the population.

Current individual based simulation models of STD transmission allow us to explore the relationship between sexual behavior parameters and the risk of STD infection, both for the individual and for the population. The influence of such parameters is likely to differ according to both the biology of the particular STD and the stage of an infection's history within a population. The importance of "concurrent" connections in the sexual partner network is twofold. First, the breaks in transmission chains if partnerships do not occur in the "correct" order are avoided, but perhaps more importantly, concurrency avoids a waiting time between infection and new partnership formation. In the case of acute bacterial STDs this waiting time could provide opportunities for recovery. Thus, concurrency makes it more likely that a bacterial STD will persist. Whereas, with viral STDs which have a long duration of infectiousness a waiting time would slow down the epidemic spread of infection. In this case concurrency speeds the growth of epidemics, but the cumulative number of partners of those infected is likely to be more important to the endemic prevalence or final size of an epidemic than whether those partnerships coexist in time. The importance of "concurrent" partnerships in such situations also depends upon the characteristics of what is described as concurrent behavior—the frequency and timing of the acts within the partnerships becomes important to the opportunities for and timing of transmission. Thus, while it is clear that network parameters influence STD epidemiology more consideration should be given to the definition of these parameters and their interrelationship.

Using individual based simulation models (Ghani et al. 1997; Ghani and Garnett 2000) have explored the sensitivity of a bacterial infection to a range of parameters describing the sexual partner networks. The results of these analyses make intuitive sense: the persistence of infection is controlled by the presence of chains of infection, thus, the proportion of the population in mutually (for whatever reason) nonmonogamous relationships, and the interconnectedness of those with many partners were the most significant determinants of persistence. Beyond persistence prevalence is dominated by how large a fraction of the population are in contact with what could be termed the "core group." Thus, the partner choice of those within the high activity, coherent part of the sex partner network was the most significant determinant of prevalence (Ghani et al. 1997). A similar logistic regression analysis of infection of individuals in simulations of the transmission of a bacterial STD in a sex partner network explored the influence of parameters describing their position within the sexual network. The most important risk factor was the number of sex partners, followed by "concurrency" and partners' number of partners. However, a range of measures of global centrality carried additional predictive power when combined with these measures of local centrality. Interestingly, when comparing the risk of acquiring versus transmitting infection the importance of concurrency was greater in the risk of transmitting infection where the propagation of infection is more likely if one can be infected and immediately transmit infection to an existing partner (Ghani and Garnett 2000).

6.6.6 Implications for STD prevention

Mixing patterns, partnership types, and partner characteristics influence many aspects of STD prevention. Information about local and global networks, and mixing patterns may facilitate sexual risk assessment and may enable STD programs to better target their prevention efforts. Partner notification, a cornerstone of STD control, is particularly influenced by partnership types, partner characteristics, and mixing patterns.

In an effort to evaluate the demographic and behavioral characteristics of STD patients and their partners that predict success in partner notification efforts, we analyzed Stage I data from interviews with 225 heterosexual patients with gonorrhea or chlamydial infection who received care at the STD clinic or at other facilities in Seattle-King County (Whittington et al. 1995). Patients reported 412 sexual partnerships during the 90-day period prior to diagnosis. Patient characteristics associated with failure to locate and refer sex partners included minority race/ethnicity, and multiple sex partners; diagnosis (gonorrhea versus chlamydia) and source of health care (public versus private) were not associated with partner referral success. Sex partner characteristics associated with unsuccessful referral included: multiple sex partners, sex worker, and among male sex partners, carrying an electronic pager. Persons involved in sexual partnerships of <90 days duration were less likely to be successfully referred than were partners in longer duration relationships. Markers of access to the partner, including knowledge of phone number or address, were all associated with successful referral.

To better understand patients' perceptions of partner notification and how their motivations for notifying their partners are related to partnership types, we analyzed data from Stage II in-depth interviews with sixty heterosexual men and women with gonorrhea, chlamydia, or nongonococcal urethritis and nineteen MSM with gonorrhea. We found that notifying the main partner was the typical pattern. Least likely to be notified were MSM's oral sex and anonymous contacts; men's one time partners; women's incarcerated and former partners; and for all groups partners perceived as transmitters, and partners who preceded onset of symptoms. People had a variety of reasons for not notifying their partners: young heterosexuals feared gossip, women feared violence, and MSM feared rejection (Tables 6.1 and 6.2; Gorbach et al. 2000).

An ongoing study of partner notification in Seattle (Stage IV) builds on previous research to use sexual network data to direct and evaluate a gonorrhea and chlamydia prevention intervention. In September of 1998 we expanded PN services in Seattle to affect people diagnosed with gonorrhea or chlamydial infection outside of public health STD clinics. As part of this expansion of service, we instituted a randomized trial comparing different types of PN, the Partners Study. This study also collects egocentric network data. At present, the study enrolls 25 percent of all English-speaking, nonincarcerated heterosexuals over age 13 diagnosed with gonorrhea or chlamydial infection in Seattle-King County. The Partners Study randomizes patients to either standard or expedited partner care. Standard care is the traditional routine: patients are advised to refer their partners to a healthcare provider for an

Table 6.1. *Reasons To Not Notify: Quotations*

Reason	Quote	Age	Sex	Sexual partners	Ethnicity	Diagnosis
Perceived transmitter	"I got it, and somebody didn't tell me."	21	M	Opposite sex	AA	Non-gonoccal urethritis
	"…the bottom line is that it was pretty clear to me that he communicated that disease to me. Where HE got it I don't know. But I guess I thought he is going to discover it and if he does not already know that he has it, he will."	35	M	Same sex	Caucasian	Gonorrhea
	"It be like anytime I have gotten an STD, it has been with somebody on the side. They didn't tell me, I ain't going to tell them."	16	F	Opposite sex	AA	Chlamydial infection
Fear of gossip	"I'm not going to tell no one because then it would be embarrassing on me they would tell everybody else and I don't want to be known as having no STDs."	19	M	Opposite sex	AA	Gonorrhea
	"No, I figured they would go tell. That would be the talk of Seattle for me."	15	F	Opposite sex	AA	Chlamydial infection
Fear of abuse	"I'm too scared too. Honestly, I'm too scared. D— told me so I confirmed it with him. I said I can't tell anyone else and he said they will call for you and I said no, no…I think I know where I got it from. There were three guys…I'm too scared."	21	F	Opposite sex	Caucasian	Chlamydial infection
	"…After he found out it was really true he would come after me…he gets angry and says you better look out or I'm going to hit you…"	16	F	Opposite sex	AA	Chlamydial infection
Fear of rejection	"Ah, not unless they asked me. Just because they would, um if you had an STD they would forget you…fear of them not wanting me."	28	M	Same sex	Caucasian	Gonorrhea

Table 6.2. *Quotations of Patients' Notification Choices*

Notify	Quote of why notify partners	Age	Gender R	Gender P	Ethnic group	STD
All	"I did not feel uncomfortable. I did for a second knowing I would have to call them. But it was not like they were people that I really knew so, I think that would have been more uncomfortable. Somebody I had known for a long time that I had started dating—that would be devastating. Cause of the fear that they are going to leave you or something or hate you…"	34	M	M	Caucasian	GC
	"I would rather tell somebody and have them check and not find it than not tell somebody who has it and is spreading it further. But I did not want to run the risk of it spreading…So I contacted three people, oh four guys…"	48	M	M	Caucasian	GC
	"…I do it because I care about people more than just a roll in the hay."	35	M	F	AA	CT
Only	"I know what goes on with him and he knows what goes on with me. If I don't feel like I could trust him I wouldn't tell him about the herpes I would just tell him I had a yeast infection."	18	F	M	AA	GC
	"My girlfriend was fine, I mean she pretty much expected it from me, she knows all about my past…"	21	M	F	F	CT
	"I didn't want to make it seem that it was all my fault so I said I found out that I have chlamydia and I think you need to get checked up. I don't know who gave it to whom because we both have unprotected sex sometimes so you can't really point the finger. That way they can't be mad…"	17	F	M	AA	CT
Main not others	"You tell the most important person and the other ones, they can find out on their own. You don't care nothing about them no way. The ones you don't care about are the ones that run their mouth and you don't want your business all out on the street."	16	F	M	AA	CT

Table 6.2. (*Continued*)

Notify	Quote of why notify partners	Age	Gender R	Gender P	Ethnic group	STD
	"I told my fiancé. I didn't tell no one else because I figured it wasn't any of their business...I only wanted to tell my fiancé."	19	M	F	AA	CT
	"Obviously my primary partner knew because he had it first. And if I had it first I would have told him. I have not yet talked with the other person but I do want to tell him, the one person. And the other person I don't really even have a way of getting in touch with him unless I recognize him on the board"	31	M	M	Caucasian	GC
Others not main	"I contacted one, my primary partner was out of town so I did not have to worry about that at all. So I contacted three people, oh four guys... my main primary partner does not know I had it."	48	M	M	Caucasian	GC
Some, not others	"...at the time there were pretty much, like four potential people before, I mean I kind of thought it was one of two but there were four and two of them I had phone numbers for, two of them I had no idea who they were, where they were so...And the two of them, you know, I gave to the clinic lady and said 'you go ahead and do it'..."	26	M	M	Caucasian	GC
	"No, I didn't (tell anyone else) because I haven't been with anyone else since I started to have symptoms..."	19	M	F	AA	CT
	"I will probably tell him, but I'll, the thing is that...we didn't have any anal sex in the park...but I don't think he's gonna show anything because, I mean we had sex, we did oral sex but I don't think he could catch it from oral sex, I don't think you can catch it by oral sex..."	26	M	M	AA	GC
None	"...Because I didn't want to break things up even more than we have already...".	24	M	F	NA	GC

Table 6.2. *(Continued)*

Notify	Quote of why notify partners	Age	Gender R	Gender P	Ethnic group	STD
	"I didn't tell (that) lady, no, because I wasn't talking to her no more at that point. There were some other partners in the same general time period but I didn't call them up neither because... I wasn't actually having sex at the same time I was with her. There was no way it could get from me to them."	44	M	F	AA	CT
	"There was one other sex partner, and we didn't actually talk about it, but I think she knew and got treated..."	21	M	F	F	CT
	"I am not going to tell no one. I hope they all get some too because it was from one of them."	19	M	F	AA	GC

Note: GC, gonorrhea; CT, chlamydia.

STD examination and treatment. Expedited management involves direct, no-cost treatment of partners without prior clinical examination, a strategy employed by many health care providers but of uncertain efficacy. A novel aspect of the study is that most medication is distributed through collaboration with commercial pharmacies. The study's primary endpoint is prevalence of infection 10–18 weeks after treatment. This is an individual measure of prevention efficacy.

In order to assess the intervention's prevention impact at the population level, we propose to use sexual network data to estimate the impact of the intervention on disease prevalence. Network data will be used to parameterize an individual based stochastic model of gonorrhea and chlamydial transmission. The necessity to represent multiple ongoing partnerships with a finite duration is a consequence of the outcome measure of reinfection and provides a more appropriate description of the actual epidemiology of STIs. To date, work on modeling such networks has concentrated on the parameters which determine the incidence of infection at the individual and population level and the biases in their measurement (Ghani et al. 1997; Ghani and Garnett 1998; Ghani et al. 1998). The proposed modeling will extend this work to explore the impact of interventions in a similar manner to that employed by Kretzschmar and Morris (1996) but firmly basing scenarios and consequent cost effectiveness analyses on the results of the trial (Kretzschmar and Morris 1996).

6.7 CONCLUSIONS

Over the past decade our understanding of how mixing patterns, network characteristics, temporal ordering of sex partnerships, and types of sex partnerships affect the spread of STI has been enhanced greatly. However, the list of unresolved issues and unanswered research questions is lengthy indeed. In what follows we briefly list some of these problems. It is important to have future research attention focus on these issues.

In STD clinic settings elicitation of names of sex partners carries both research and program significance. Improvement of the efficacy of name elicitation techniques is of great importance and would help further both research and program goals. In many cases STD spread rapidly through sexual interactions between persons who do not know each other's names. Even in such situations network approaches may be partially applicable and helpful by shifting attention from elicitation of names to identification of places where partners are met and where sex takes place; or to description of partners demographic, social, and behavioral characteristics. Techniques that could be applied in situations of "anonymous sex" need to be described.

The importance of the parameters describing sex partner networks in STD transmission is becoming better established. However, the biases in estimation of these parameters poses a serious problem since it is unlikely that complete unbiased measurement will ever be possible (Ghani and Garnett 1998*b*; Ghani et al. 1998*a*). The simulation of sampling methods should be able to contribute to improving study design. Further work is required to explore the role of the network for particular infections at particular phases of STD epidemics (Wasserheit and Aral 1996). Modeling efforts that help explain the mechanism of action of different network patterns in increasing or decreasing the rate of spread of STD need to be continued. It is important to understand how mixing patterns and networks affect STD transmission dynamics, and to employ such understanding in the development of interventions for STD prevention.

It is clear that distinct mixing patterns, network structures, and partnership types emerge in response to broader social, economic, demographic, and cultural factors. Future research should identify these determinants and explore ways of preventing the formation of mixing patterns, network structures, and partnership types that are highly conducive to rapid spread of STI.

References

Aral, S., Holmes, K. et al. (1996). "Overview: Individual and population approaches to the epidemiology and prevention of sexually transmitted diseases and human immunodeficiency virus infection," *J Infect Dis*, 174(Suppl 2): S127–33.
—— Hughes, J. et al. (1994). "Demographic and behavioral concordance between sex partners: Partnerships infected with chlamydia trachomatis are different than those infected with gonorrhea and syphilis." *Chlamydial Infections: Proceedings of the Eighth International Symposium on Human Chlamydial Infections*. Chantilly, France, 19–24 Bologna, Italy: Societa Editrice Esculapio.
—— —— et al. (1995). Demographic and behavioral concordance between sex partners: Effects of demographic and partnership characteristics, sexual behavior and infection status. Presented at the IUVDT Regional Meetings, Singapore.

—— —— et al. (1998). "The spread of chlamydial infection: Sexual mixing patterns, infection rates, linked morbidities, and bridge populations in Seattle, Washington." In G. I. Byrne, G. Christiansen, I. N. Clarke et al. (eds.), *Chlamydial Infections: Proceedings of the Ninth International Symposium on Human Chlamydial Infection. International Chlamydial Symposium*, pp. 19–22.

—— —— et al. (1999). "Sexual mixing patterns in the spread of gonococcal and chlamydial infections," *Am J Public Health*, 86(6): 825–33.

Bearman, P., Moody, J. et al. (2004). "Chains of affection: The structure of adolescent romantic and sexual networks." *American Journal of Sociology* (in press).

Brunham, R. and Plummer, F. A. (1990). "A general model of sexually transmitted disease epidemiology and its implications for control," *Med Clin N Am*, 74: 1339–52.

Burstein, G., Caydos, C. et al. (1998). "Incident chlamydia trachomatis infections among inner-city adolescent females," *J Am Med Assoc*, 280(6): 521–6.

Catania, J., Binson, D. et al. (1995). "Risk factors for HIV and other sexually transmitted diseases and prevention practices among US heterosexual adults: Changes from 1990 to 1992," *Am J Public Health*, 85(11): 1492–9.

Diez-Roux, A. V. (1998). "Bringing context back into epidemiology: Variables and fallacies in multilevel analysis," *Am J Public Health*, 88(2): 216–22.

Foxman, B. and Holmes, K. K. (1995). Partnership characteristics is a general population: Final technical report submitted to DSTDP, CDC.

—— Aral, S. et al. (1998). "Interrelationships among douching practices, risk sexual practices, and history of self-reported sexually transmitted diseases in an urban population," *Sex Transm Dis*, 25: 90–9.

Garnett, G. and Anderson, R. (1993). "Contact tracing and the estimation of sexual mixing patterns: The epidemiology of gonococcal infections," *Sex Transm Dis*, 20(4): 181–91.

—— Hughes, J. et al. (1996). "Sexual mixing patterns of patients attending sexually transmitted diseases clinics," *Sex Transm Dis*, 23(3): 248–57.

Ghani, A., Donnelly, C. et al. (1998). "Sampling biases and missing data in explorations of sexual partner networks for the spread of sexually transmitted diseases," *Stat Med*, 17(18): 2079–97.

—— and Garnett, G. (1998). "Measuring sexual partner networks for STD transmission," *J R Stat Soc A*, 161: 227–38.

—— —— (2000). "The risk of acquiring and transmitting infection in sexual partner networks," *Sex Transm Dis*, 27(10): 579–87.

Ghani, A. C., Swinton, J. et al. (1997). "The role of sexual partnership networks in the epidemiology of gonorrhea," *Sex Trans Dis*, 24(1): 45–56.

Gorbach, P., Aral, S. et al. (2000). "It takes a village: The need for concurrent sexual partnerships in Seattle, WA." Presented at the STI at the Millennium—Past, Present, and Future: The First Joint MSSVD—ASTDA Conference, Baltimore, MD, May 3–6.

—— —— et al. (2000). "To notify or not to notify: STD patients' perspectives of partner notification in Seattle sexually transmitted diseases," *Sex Transm Dis*, 27(4): 193–200.

—— Stoner, B. et al. (1997). "Sleeping around in Seattle: A qualitative assessment of sexual partnerships." Poster at the International Conference for Sexually Transmitted Disease Research, Seville, Spain, October 19–21.

Granath, F., Giesecke, J. et al. (1991). "Estimation of a preference matrix for women's choice of male sexual partner according to rate of partner change using partner notification data," *Math Biosc*, 107: 341–8.

Gupta, S. and Anderson, R. M. (1989). "Networks of sexual contacts: Implications for the pattern of spread of HIV," *AIDS*, 3: 807–17.

Hsu Schmitz, S. and Castillo-Chavez, C. (1994). "Parameter estimation in non-closed social networks related to dynamics of sexually transmitted diseases." In E. Kaplan and M. Brandeau (eds.), *Modeling the AIDS Epidemic.* New York: Raven Press.

Joyner, K., Carver, K. et al. (1998). "Adolescent dating and romantic relationships." Paper presented at the Population Association of America Meetings, Chicago, IL.

Kretzschmar, M. and Morris, M. (1996). "Measures of concurrency in networks and the spread of infectious disease," *Math Biosc,* 133: 165–95.

Laumann, E., Gagnon, J. et al. (1994). *The Social Organization of Sexuality: Sexual Practices in the United States.* Chicago, IL: The University of Chicago Press.

Liang, K. and Zeger, S. (1986). "Longitudinal data analysis using generalized linear models," *Biometrika,* 73: 13–22.

Lin, L. (1989). "A concordance correlation coefficient to evaluate reproducibility," *Biometrics,* 45: 255–68.

Manhart, L. E., Aral, S. O., Holmes K. K., and Foxman, B. (2002). "Sex partner concurrency—measurement, prevalence and correlates among urban 18–39 year olds," *Sex Transm Dis,* 29(3): 133–43.

Morris, M. (1991). "A log-linear modeling framework for selective mixing," *Math Biosc,* 107: 349–77.

——and Dean, L. (1994). "The effects of sexual behavior change on long-term HIV seroprevalence among homosexual men," *Am J Epidemiol,* 140(3): 217–32.

——and Kretzschmar, M. (1997). "Concurrent partnerships and the spread of HIV," *AIDS,* 11: 641–8.

Padian, N., Aral, S. et al. (1996). "Individual and population approaches to the epidemiology and prevention of sexually transmitted diseases and human immunodeficiency virus infection," *J Infect Dis,* 174(Suppl): S1227–57.

Potterat, J. J., Rothenberg, R. B. et al. (1985). "Gonorrhoea as a social disease," *Sex Transm Dis,* 12: 25–32.

Rothenberg, R. B. (1983). "The geography of gonorrhea: Empirical demonstration of core group transmission," *Am J Epidemiol,* 117: 688–94.

Ryan, C., Courtois, B. et al. (1998). "Risk assessment, symptoms, and signs as predictors of vulvovaginal and cervical infections in an urban US STD clinic: Implications for use of STD algorithms," *Sex Trans Infect,* 74(Suppl 1): S59–76.

Service, S. and Blower, S. (1995). "HIV transmission in sexual networks: an empirical analysis," *Proc R Soc Lond B Biol Sci,* 260(1359): 237–44.

————(1996). "Linked HIV epidemics in San Francisco (letter to the editor)," *J AIDS and Hum Retrovirol,* 2: 1–2.

Sonenstein, F., Ku, L. et al. (1998). "Changes in sexual behavior and condom use among teenaged males: 1988 to 1995," *Am J Public Health,* 88: 956–9.

Stoner, B., Whittington, W. et al. (1993). "Variation in frequency of sex partner change within sexually transmitted disease networks". Program and abstracts of the 33rd Interscience Conference on Antimicrobial Agents and Chemotherapy (ICACC), p. 119.

————(1997). "Sociometric validation of sex partner risk assessment." Abstracts of the 12th Meeting of the International Society for STD Research (ISSTDR), Seville, Spain.

————(2000). "Comparative epidemiology of heterosexual gonococcal and chlamydial networks: Implications for transmission patterns," *Sex Transm Dis,* 27(4): 215–23.

————(2003). "Avoiding risky sex partners: Perception of partners' risk v. partners' self reported risks," *Sex Transm Infect,* 79(3): 197–201.

Sturm, A., Wilkinson, D. et al. (1998). "Pregnant women as a reservoir of undetected sexually transmitted diseases in rural South Africa: Implications for disease control," *Am J Public Health*, 88(8): 1243–5.

Taha, E., Canner, J. K. et al. (1996). "Reported condom use is not associated with incidence of sexually transmitted diseases in Malawi," *AIDS*, 10: 207–12.

Thomas, J., Kulik, A. et al. (1995). "Syphilis in the south: Rural rates surpass urban rates in North Carolina," *Am J Public Health*, 85(8): 1119–21.

Turnbull, B. (1976). "The empirical distribution function with arbitrarily grouped, censored and truncated data," *J Royal Stat Soc Ser B*, 38: 290–5.

Turner, C., Ku, L. et al. (1998). "Adolescent sexual behavior, drug use, and violence: Increased reporting with computer survey technology," *Science*, May(280): 5365.

Wasserheit, J. and Aral, S. (1996). "The dynamic topology of sexually transmitted disease epidemics: Implications for prevention strategies c," *J Infect Dis*, 174(Suppl 2): S201–13.

Whittington, W., Stoner, B. et al. (1995). "Correlates of success in sex partner referral and evaluation among persons with gonococcal or chlamydial infection." Abstracts of the 11th Meeting of the International Society for STD Research (ISSTDR), p. 223.

Zenilman, J., Bonner, M. et al. (1988). "Penicillinase-producing Neisseria gonorrhoeae in Dade County, Florida: Evidence of core-group transmitters and the impact of illicit antibiotics," *Sex Trans Dis*, 15(1): 45–50.

PART III

COMPLETE NETWORK DESIGNS

7

The Collection and Analysis of Social Network Data in Nang Rong, Thailand

RONALD R. RINDFUSS, AREE JAMPAKLAY,
BARBARA ENTWISLE, YOTHIN SAWANGDEE,
KATHERINE FAUST, AND PRAMOTE PRASARTKUL

7.1 INTRODUCTION

In recent years, interest in social network approaches has increased substantially. Undoubtedly AIDS, with its intrinsic network aspects and inevitable fatal outcome, was the largest single contributor to this renewed interest in aspects of social networks among researchers interested in population and health issues. However, social network interest has also been generated among social demographers examining migration and fertility. Among migration researchers, social networks can provide crucial links between places of origin and potential destinations (e.g. Massey et al. 1987; Boyd 1989). Among fertility researchers, concerns with the evaluation of family planning programs along with the diffusion of ideas, information, and methods have led to considerable research using social network ideas, data, and methods (e.g. Watkins 1991; Kincaid et al. 1993; Montgomery and Casterline 1993; Jato et al. 1995; Mita and Simmons 1995; Entwisle et al. 1996). Indeed this interest has led to re-analyses of the data collected in Korea in the 1960s that linked social networks and reproductive behavior (Chung 1993; Valente 1995; Kohler 1997). Until recently, this rich Korean data had not been fully exploited.

In this chapter we describe our experiences collecting and analyzing social network data as part of a longitudinal study of general social and demographic

The work reported in this chapter is part of a larger set of interrelated projects. Funding support for the set of projects includes grants from the National Institute of Child Health and Human Development (RO1-HD33570, R01 HD37896, and RO1-HD25482), The National Science Foundation (SBR 93-10366), The Evaluation Project (USAID Contract #DPE-3060-C-00-1054), The MEASURE Project, the National Aeronautic and Space Administration, and the MacArthur Foundation (95-31576A-POP). The larger set of projects involves various collaborations between investigators at the Carolina Population Center (CPC), University of North Carolina and the Institute for Population and Social Research (IPSR), Mahidol University, including Aphichat Chamratrithirong, Chanya Sethaput, Kanchana Tangchonlatip, Thirapong Santiphot, and Stephen Walsh. Expert programming and spatial analysis assistance has been provided by Rick O'Hara, Phil Page, Alan Snavely, Erika Stone, John Vogler, and Karin Willert. Peter Bearman and Sara Curran provided substantial input into the design of the social network questions.

change in Nang Rong, Thailand. This longitudinal study began in 1984—prior to the recent revival of interest in social networks within the population field. Thus our motivation was not to do a social network study, but rather to add a network component to an ongoing study of social and economic change. While not directly concerned with the spread of AIDS or other infectious diseases, our experiences have relevance for those with such interests. For example, we obtain geographic coordinates for actors in social networks. This allows a geographic visualization of social network properties. It also permits comparison of social and geographic distance. The extension of this geographic-social network to disease models is a logical next step for those who study the transmission of AIDS and other infectious diseases. One could examine the spatial patterning of a disease in conjunction with the spatial pattern of social networks. Another example is our successful follow-up of out-migrants using known properties of social networks in our study area. Similar issues are likely to arise in attempting to trace sexual partners. In short, in the language of social networks, in the context of this volume, our chapter is a "bridge" chapter, linking ongoing efforts in the fertility and migration fields with those in the AIDS and infectious diseases fields. To date, our project has not specifically addressed the AIDS issue.

7.2 STUDY LOCATION: NANG RONG, THAILAND

To understand the nature and potential of the social network data we have collected, it is important to know key features of Nang Rong, our study site. These include size, economy, spatial organization, demographic history, and tradition of cooperation.

Nang Rong district is located in Buriram province, in Northeast Thailand (see Map 7.1). The district is relatively small spatially, approximately 1300 square kilometers, about the size of an Eastern US county. It is also relatively small from a demographic perspective, containing 183,000 people in 1990 (National Statistics Office 1990). There were 310 rural villages in 1994 plus several market/administrative towns. Villages average about 100 households. Given this, saturated as opposed to ego-based networks are thinkable, both among households within villages and among villages within the district.

Nang Rong district is part of an area known as Isaan. Agriculture, especially rice cultivation, dominates the local economy. This area is among the poorest in Thailand, largely because of poor soils combined with low and unstable rainfall (Parnwell 1988). Over 80 percent of the average annual rain occurs during May to September, with soil moisture deficits common at other times (Rigg 1991). Floods and droughts are frequent (Fukui 1993). This means that households need to diversify risk, and a common approach is seasonal migration during the dry season. Households have network links to a number of places outside Nang Rong by virtue of migrant flows.

Within the Nang Rong villages, dwelling units are organized in a cluster, surrounded by agricultural land. Residents of the village know one another. The typical household uses two or three parcels of land, and these parcels tend not to be contiguous with one

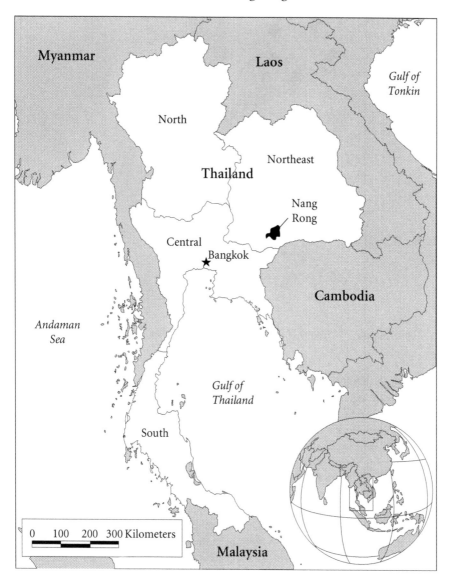

Map 7.1. *Study Area Location, Nang Rong District, Northeast Thailand*

another. (See Fig. 7.1 for an illustration.) The parcels are fairly small and most agriculture in the district is rain fed rather than irrigated. This means that most households engaged in farming activities are dependent on the annual monsoon for the timing of the agricultural season and are likely to be engaged in agricultural activities at the same time as other households. Agricultural activities are occurring on small plots about the

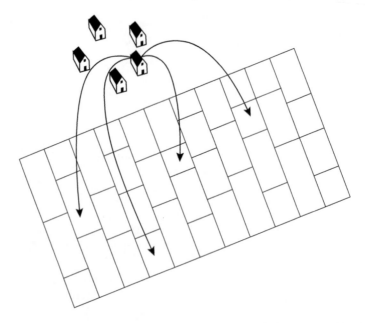

Figure 7.1. *An Illustration of Nucleated Villages with Households Using Multiple Plots*

same time so that interactions are also likely taking place during periods of field preparation, planting, transplanting, weeding, and harvesting.

The demographic history of the district is such that young adults now have unusually large numbers of living siblings. Those who were in their 20s and early 30s during the 1994/5 round of data collection were born after mortality had declined (and hence significantly more infants were surviving to adulthood) but before (or during) the time when fertility was declining. Thus, with large numbers being born and experiencing increased survival chances, the number of siblings is unusually large, and siblings are likely to have a more important role in each other's lives.

Finally, it should be noted that Thais in general are very cooperative with social science researchers, certainly more so than in the United States, and possibly more so than in many countries. Within Thailand, rural households are more cooperative than urban ones. During data collection times, our interviewers actually live in the villages where they are collecting data. They are known to members of the community and become trusted. The result is a remarkably high level of cooperation.

7.3 SAMPLE

The Nang Rong Surveys began as an evaluation. In 1984, the Population and Community Development Association (PDA) began a Community Based Integrated Rural Development (CBIRD) project in selected villages in Nang Rong district. The CBIRD project was designed to (*a*) improve skills and productive capacity in agriculture, animal husbandry, and various cottage industries, such as raising silk worms, and (*b*) upgrade waste disposal facilities, increase year-round availability of drinking water, and promote health practices. PDA asked the Institute for Population and Social Research (IPSR) at Mahidol University to evaluate the success of the CBIRD project. IPSR designed and conducted a multilevel baseline survey in 1984. First, fifty villages were chosen. These were divided into forty villages chosen to receive the benefits of the CBIRD project (project villages) and ten that were to be non-project or control villages. By the time the fieldwork began one of the villages had administratively split into two, and so the number of villages in 1984 was fifty-one.

Once the CBIRD project began, it became clear that the idea of having control or non-project villages was not practical. People from the non-project villages stopped at CBIRD headquarters. Project and non-project villages interacted with one another. Hence, the distinction between project and non-project villages was dropped.[1]

Community surveys[2] were conducted in these fifty-one villages, followed by a complete household census. The census obtained information on all household members. The 1984 round was not designed as a social network study, but its design lent itself to including network components. As is typical in surveys in rural Thailand conducted by university-based social scientists, the response rates were excellent. Nonresponse was such a non-issue that information was not kept on how many households refused. However, talking with those who were part of the staff in 1984, including interviewers, suggests that response rates were well in excess of 90 percent, and likely over 99 percent.[3]

The initial collaboration between the Carolina Population Center (CPC) and IPSR, which began after the 1984 data collection, focused on contraceptive use. The collaboration was subsequently broadened to include social networks, migration, and the environment. An expanded data collection took place in 1994/95, building on the earlier surveys and also reflecting these new interests.[4] The 1994/95 data collection was the first time social network approaches were included in the Nang Rong longitudinal data sets. We describe this 1994/95 data collection in some detail, with particular emphasis on the collection of social network data.

There are three components to the 1994/95 data collection: A household survey, a migrant follow-up, and a community profile. Figure 7.2 shows how they interrelate, with each other and also with the 1984 and (planned[5]) 2000 surveys.

---

[1] In our multivariate analyses on a variety of topics we have tested for differences between project and non-project villages. We have not found it to be important, and so for all practical purposes we treat the two sets of villages in a similar fashion.

[2] The community surveys obtained contextual data for each village, including information on agricultural technology, electricity, and various social institutions.

[3] Asking interviewers or supervisors about refusals usually brings a puzzled look to their face. If they think about it long enough, they might remember an occasion when a household refused. However, all the evidence is consistent with remarkably high response rates.

[4] Between 1984 and 1988 there were a variety of small-scale data collection efforts aimed at answering specific and specialized questions. But there was no large-scale effort between 1984 and 1994/95.

[5] Between the time this chapter was written and its publication, the 2000 data collection occurred successfully. The final section of this chapter provides a brief description.

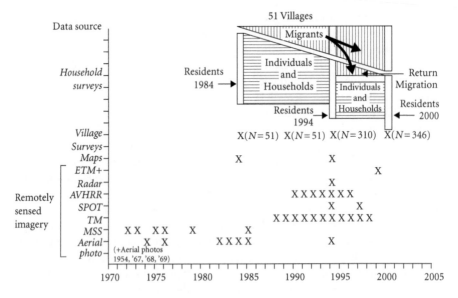

Figure 7.2. *Nang Rong Data*

The 1994 Household Survey was a complete census of all households in each of the fifty-one villages in the 1984 survey. Again cooperation was excellent, resulting in near universal coverage of all households in the fifty-one villages, and again exact response rates are not available. Data were collected between April and July 1994 from 7337 households. Information was obtained on 42,219 current and former members of these households.

An innovative feature of the 1994 round of data collection was the tracking and interviewing of migrants—individuals or households that were present in 1984 but were not present in 1994. The 1994/5 Migrant Follow-up collected data from out-migrants from twenty-two of the original fifty-one villages. Persons resident in 1984 but no longer resident in 1994 were candidates for follow-up if they had migrated to one of four destinations: Metropolitan Bangkok; the Eastern Seaboard (a focus of rapid growth and development), Korat (a regional city), or Buriram (the provincial capital). Migrants can be linked to their 1984 origin household, the successor to that household in 1994, and (at least in a limited way) to other migrants from the village.

The migrant survey began in September 1994 and continued through May 1995. Almost 1900 migrants were interviewed. Calculating follow-up rates is difficult for several reasons. First, for many migrants origin households did not know where they were, and hence we cannot be sure of the correct denominators. Our fieldwork procedures incorporated social network features. Whenever we found a migrant, we would show that migrant a list of migrants from her or his village and ask if they knew the whereabouts of any of them. If they did and we had not yet interviewed them, we would attempt to do so. This resulted in our interviewing some migrants who were in our destination locations, but this was not reported by the origin house-holds. There were also situations when the origin household reported they were in a non-target destination, and we actually found and interviewed them in a target destination. This could happen because they had moved between the time of the field-work in the fifty-one villages and the migrant follow-up fieldwork. Or it could simply be the case that the origin household was misinformed. The details of the follow-up rates are reported elsewhere (Rindfuss, Kaneda et al. 2003). But, in general, given the difficulty in following migrants after ten years, the fieldwork went remarkably well.

There is one final comment we would like to make about the design of the migrant follow-up. Originally, we planned to find and interview migrants in their places of des-tination, but it became clear that this was a difficult, time-consuming, and expensive strategy. During the migrant fieldwork we began to interview migrants in their home villages when they returned for holidays (New Year, Chinese New Year, Songkran) and this turned out to be cost-effective. More than a quarter of the migrant interviews occurred in the origin villages.

The third and final component of the 1994/95 data collection was the community survey. Interviews were conducted between March and June 1994. Information was col-lected about the size and composition of the village, cropping patterns, water sources, agricultural technology, electrification, transportation and communication, health and family planning services, village groups and committees, and perceptions about defor-estation. In contrast to the 1984 community survey, which focused on the same fifty-one villages included in the household survey, the 1994 community survey covered all villages in Nang Rong district (310), including but not limited to the original fifty-one.

For all phases of the fieldwork, small gifts were given to respondents. These were not meant as inducements to participate. Rather they were meant as a way to say thank you for participating. For example, in the household interview, respondents were given a plastic shopping bag decorated with elephants (with elephants symbol-izing the magnitude of the data collection undertaking).

7.4 DATA COLLECTION AND MANAGEMENT

7.4.1 *Questionnaire design*

The actual questionnaires used in the interviewing can be found on our web site, www.cpc.unc.edu/projects/nangrong/nangrong_home.html, both in Thai and English. Here we simply provide an overview, beginning with the household ques-tionnaires. They obtained social and demographic facts about current members; yearly life history data for those between 18 and 35, including information about work and migration patterns; sibling ties for those between 18 and 35; household characteristics, including plots of land owned and rented, use of agricultural equip-ment, crop mix, planting and harvesting of rice, cassava, and sugar cane, which rice mill the household used, and household debts; the whereabouts and current charac-teristics of 1984 household members no longer residing in the household; and visits and exchanges of goods and money with former household members.

An innovative feature of the household survey was the collection of complete household networks within villages. Using a household list obtained from village headmen and updated as needed during the course of the fieldwork, ties to other households in the village due to sibling relationships, help with the most recent rice harvest, and the renting, hiring, and sharing of agricultural equipment (tractors and water pumps) were coded.[6] With data for complete household networks in fifty-one villages, it is possible to compare networks across those fifty-one villages. For ties outside of the village, we coded the village number if the village was in Nang Rong district, the district number if the link was outside Nang Rong district but in Buriram Province, and the province number otherwise. The availability of information on ties to other villages makes it possible to investigate the salience of village boundaries to the network structure. We need not assume that social networks within villages are closed. Information about membership in the most active local group (determined as part of the village survey, which preceded household data collection), where household members lived at age 10, and use of local rice mills was also collected in the household survey—information that can be used to infer social networks. A complete list of specific questions included in the household survey that are relevant to social networks is contained in the Appendix to this chapter.

The migrant follow-up obtained information about actual migration experience, contact with other migrants from the origin village, visits and exchanges of goods and money with the origin household in Nang Rong, yearly life history data for the migrant and for others between 18 and 35 living in the migrant's household, sibling ties, and household characteristics. A substantial amount of social network data was collected, including some ego-based questions about potential help finding a job or borrowing money in the place of destination. The Appendix lists the specific questions included in the Migrant Follow-up.

The community questionnaire also contained social network information. Complete networks based on sharing temples, schools, water sources, bus routes, and access to major highways as well as those arising directly from labor exchanges and equipment rental are part of the village data. One can also consider ties outside Nang Rong district. By design, the household network data are embedded within village networks. Thus, social ties can be viewed from a multilevel perspective. The Appendix lists the social network generators included in the village survey.

All the questionnaires were interviewer administered, typically in a group setting. For example, in the household interviews, frequently multiple members of the household were present, and sometimes neighbors. Since we did not ask any sensitive questions or attitudinal items, this group interview approach worked quite well. Frequently, if the primary respondent did not know the answer to a question, another household member would supply the information. Further, the group interview approach also made the participants feel more comfortable and relaxed.

---

[6] The design of these questions was based on prior qualitative fieldwork, which suggested that considerable social interaction occurred while women were milling rice and while members of different households were helping each other with agricultural activities.

7.4.2 Fieldwork

During the fieldwork in the villages, interviewers stayed in the village and got to know villagers. This developed trust between the interviewers and village residents, and thus respondents were more likely to give the interviewers the locations of migrant household members. There were seven teams of interviewers, and each team had one assistant supervisor and four or five interviewers.

Supervisors were full time researchers of IPSR. Assistant supervisors were recruited specifically for the project, in Bangkok, and they had at least a Bachelors degree. They participated in questionnaire pre-testing in Nang Rong prior to the actual fieldwork. Interviewers were recruited from Buriram province, the province where Nang Rong is located. We wanted interviewers who would be familiar with local dialects. They were recruited through contacts that IPSR had with the local teachers college (Rachapadth Institute). All had just graduated. After the interviewing was completed, some of the interviewers were retained for the data entry phase of the project.

Interviews lasted about 1 hour or so. However, there was considerable variation depending on the size and composition of the family. Once the interviewers were proficient with the intricacies of the questionnaire, length of interview was not problematic for either the respondents or the interviewers. The social network questions were among those that were the most difficult. Respondents usually needed time to think about members of the various networks. People present at the interview (not the main respondent) were often helpful recalling who helped with the rice harvest or providing information on the sibling networks of in-laws.

Perhaps the most problematic aspect of the social network data collection was using the list of all households. Consider the help with rice harvest network question. In the household surveys people were asked whether or not they planted rice in the last year. If "yes," they were asked

Q. 6.24 Did anyone from this village help to harvest rice in the last year? Record Ban Lek Ti,[7] number of people, number of days, type of labor (hire or help without pay), and the wage.

In practice, respondents remembered names of individuals, not households that helped with the rice harvest. The interviewer and the respondent then had to determine to which household that person belonged. This involved looking at the list of all households in the village, which was organized by Ban Lek Ti numbers. This entire process was facilitated because the interviewers lived in the village during the interviewing, and became quite familiar with the names of people in the village. Nevertheless, this was undoubtedly the most difficult aspect of our collection of social network data.

7.4.3 Confidentiality and the public release of data

The cost of collecting most social science data sets has escalated faster than the resources available for social science research have increased. Taking a census

---

[7] "Ban Lek Ti" can be thought of as the equivalent of a street address or apartment number. It is the number assigned to a dwelling unit by the village headman.

approach to the collection of social network data, as we have done in the 1994/95 Nang Rong survey for multiple relations and for multiple social units, is more expensive than taking an ego-based approach. Cost is one factor that has led to pressure on data collectors to make data available to the broad social science research community. Peer reviews of follow-up components of longitudinal studies typically ask about the extent to which the data have been used, both by the investigators who designed the data and also by others. The greater the use, the higher the chance that a further round of data collection will be funded. Another factor creating pressure for public release is the general utility and potential insight provided by the data. Since the days of Weber, Durkheim, and Simmel, researchers have been interested in capturing aspects of the social, physical, and ideational worlds in which individuals live their lives. Social network data speak to questions at the heart of sociology and social demography, and the relative rarity of social network data, especially linked to other information about individuals, households, and communities, only serves to increase interest in making the data public.

And yet, in potential conflict with the desirability of public release is the promise made to respondents that the information they provide will be kept confidential. Our ability to better capture the context within which individuals and households exist has increased the ability of those who wish to discover the identity of respondents to do so. Social network data are problematic in this regard. The most obvious example is a locational social network component that was being introduced in our next wave of data collection: Taking GPS readings for each household's dwelling unit. If we divulge the physical location of someone's house, we are very clearly and unequivocally releasing the identity of our respondents.

The potential for confidentiality to be breached exists even with seemingly more benign forms of social network data. Indeed, social network data are like other contextual data. Once the identity of the village (or other relatively small sampling unit) is known, it is not difficult to locate individual respondents. Consider the social network data we have for households in the Nang Rong data sets. These data feature connections between households within villages and thus provide a key to the linking of households to specific villages. In our data, once households in a particular village are identified, it is possible to identify the village by aggregating the characteristics of the households. Again, once the village is identified, respondents can also be identified. The fewer the villages, and the denser the networks within them, the easier it will be.

In short, releasing social network data of the type we have collected in Nang Rong, along with the individual and household data, is tantamount to breeching the confidentiality that was promised to respondents. We, and others involved in social science data collection, have taken the position that when there is a conflict between publicly releasing data and protecting the confidentiality of respondents that it is imperative to protect the confidentiality of respondents even if it means that a substantial amount of data is not released. We have released household and individual level data but not the social network data. We have, however, also released computed measures of household network position. While this will not satisfy all who are interested in social network analyses, it will at least satisfy the needs of some.

7.4.4 Distinctive features of the Nang Rong data from a social network perspective

What are the distinguishing features of the 1994/95 Nang Rong social network data? The most striking is that we have measured networks at multiple levels of social organization: Villages in the district, households in villages, and individual migrants. At the most general level, we have economic and social relations among the 310 villages in Nang Rong District. Then, for fifty-one villages we have census networks on kinship and economic ties. Finally, for a subset of the sampled villages, information about migrants' networks in the destination and their linkages to their origin villages were measured. It is important to note that the social units (network "actors") differ across the networks: Individual migrants, households, or villages. These are nested: Individual migrants within households, and households within villages.

For each level, multiple relations were measured. For villages, we have economic ties (movement of temporary laborers both into and out of the villages, renting large agricultural equipment—notably tractors—from other villages, and where crops are marketed), social ties (shared temples, movement of students to elementary and secondary schools), and infrastructure linkages (bus routes, road linkages, and shared water sources). At the household level, we have economic relations (help with the rice harvest and renting, hiring or sharing agricultural equipment—water pump, thresher, large tractor, tiller, or electric generator), kinship relations (sibling ties), potential social interactions (through use of the same rice mill or membership in the most important group in the village), and some information about movement between households (where people lived at age 10).

Our relations measure social or economic contact, or the potential for such contact, rather than discussion of "important" matters, or affective ties (e.g. friendship). In part this is a consequence of the kinds of units that we are studying (villages and households). Friendship or other affective ties are not well defined for these aggregate units. Also, it is theoretically and methodologically important to avoid endogeneity problems when using social network variables to understand outcomes such as contraceptive choice or migration. Had we asked people with whom they discussed contraception or migration, our ability to draw conclusions about network effects would have been severely limited. Also, our interest in social network effects has focused on the potential for the flow of information and on normative pressures on behaviors through social contacts, rather than on affective states (friendship) or perception of social support.

At both the village level and the household level our networks are census networks rather than ego-centered networks. This gives us considerable leverage to describe and model community level (rather than simply individual level) network properties. For example, we can look at households linked through indirect ties via paths including other households and we can study cohesive subsets of households in villages.

In contrast to most social network studies that are case studies of only a single group or community, we have the same measurement in numerous villages. For households in fifty-one villages and for migrants from twenty-two villages we have measured the same relations in each village. Therefore, we need not assume that all villages have the same social organization. We can compare networks across villages to see whether or not villages have similar patterns. We can also study the relationship between variation in network patterns across villages and other (non-network) characteristics of villages, such as land use.

Boundary definition is an important issue in social network studies. The problem is to delineate which actors (individuals, households, villages, or other social entities) are included in the group or community. In the Nang Rong projects our units are administratively defined (the district of Nang Rong for the village network, and the village boundaries for the household networks), but network ties might extend beyond these administrative boundaries. We can examine the extent to which social and economic relations overlap with administratively defined boundaries and the extent to which village boundaries are permeable.

7.4.5 From survey responses to social networks

Responses to the network questions in the household survey, migrant follow-up, and community questionnaires were initially recorded as variables in a SAS data file. However, there is considerable data processing involved in going from these variables to measurements of social network properties. Analyzing the social networks required constructing sociomatrices for the different relations and then calculating network properties using existing social network software (Borgatti et al. 1999) and custom written computer programs. We should note that some simple network measures, such as the number of others named on a given relation, can be calculated directly, but other network properties, such as identification of subgroups or patterns of connectedness, require the entire network or sociomatrix.

In the SAS data files, the general coding of responses to the network questions was similar for most relations, and for both household and village networks. Responses to the migrant questionnaires are more limited since the identities of those named in response to the network questions were not recorded. For the household and village networks, each relation was initially coded as a set of variables recording the identification numbers of the others (households, villages, districts, or provinces) that had been nominated in response to the question. To illustrate, consider the question in the community questionnaire that asked where residents go for temporary labor. Villages could name up to ten different locations, and hence there are ten variables. Each variable recorded the identification number of the location (the village identification number if a village in Nang Rong district was named, or the district identification number or province number if a location outside Nang Rong district was named). From these responses we constructed three sociomatrices, one with ties from villages to other villages in Nang Rong district, the second with ties from villages to other districts within the province, and the third with ties from villages to other provinces or more distant locations (i.e. abroad). The first of these sociomatrices has 310 villages as rows and 310 villages as columns. This is the sociomatrix for the village network within Nang Rong district, and was used to find network properties such as subgroups and patterns of connectedness within the village.

For household networks the procedure was similar, with two notable differences. First separate sociomatrices were constructed for each of the fifty-one villages, on each relation. Second there were four sociomatrices for each relation in each village: Ties from households to other households within the village, ties from households to villages (within Nang Rong district), ties from households to districts (within the province), and ties from households to provinces or other more distant locations (ties outside the province or abroad). For both the village and household networks, sociomatrices were then imported into a standard network analysis program or used in specially written programs to calculate network measures such as centralities, network subgroups, and network centralization.

7.4.6 Integration into Geographic Information System

The georeferencing of social networks within a Geographic Information System (GIS) is another distinguishing feature of the Nang Rong projects more generally. A GIS is an automated system for the capture, storage, retrieval, analysis, and display of spatial data (Clarke 1990). It consists of a relational database linking the geographic proportion of feature elements to their attributes and the integration of hardware, software, and geospatial information. The construction of a GIS database requires considerable investment of time and resources, and, as such, tends to only make sense when a given case or study area will be the focus of intensive research activity over a long period. We expect, however, that this will change as more spatial data becomes available in digital form and as GIS software becomes easier to use.

The starting point for the Nang Rong GIS was a set of high-quality composite maps from the early 1980s at a scale of 1:50,000, which were prepared by the Thai Ministry of Defense. We digitized these maps to create a base coverage of the study area, hydrography, transportation (including trails and foot paths), topographic contours and point elevations, village centers, market towns, and district boundaries. Building on this foundation, we subsequently added other digitized maps; additional coverages derived from the manipulation of the base coverage; aerial photographs; satellite imagery; and village characteristics (either aggregated from household data or measured in the community survey). Through the cumulation of demographic, social, economic, and environmental information over several projects, Nang Rong has become a "laboratory" for the study of social and environmental change, broadly conceived.

Social networks represented as linkages between spatially referenced points can be incorporated into a GIS database in a straightforward manner. Linkages among units of social organization located in cartographic space can be represented in this way. Thus far, our use of the GIS in social network research has focused on villages. Village locations were obtained from maps and corrected using readings taken with Global Positioning System (GPS) devices in the field. Linkage information has come largely from the 1994 community survey. Our discussion here draws on what we have learned from our work with the village networks, first presented in Faust et al. (1999). The 2000 data collection includes spatial representation of social networks at the household as well as village level. This and other features of the 2000 data collection are described later in the chapter.

The GIS serves as a key tool for integrating and analyzing data from diverse sources. Our research on village networks has combined data from the 1994 community survey; the base map (and updates from the field); and land cover classifications derived from remote images (satellite data). The flexibility of the GIS is important to inter-relating such different kinds of data. The social network and village location data are spatially discrete; information about rivers, roads, and trails is in the form of lines and polygons; and the land cover classifications are spatially continuous. While it may be obvious, it is important to note that geographic location serves as a type of ID number that permits linking information from a variety of sources.

Visual display is an important capability of the GIS. Mapping has been key to describing the spatial orientation of village networks in Nang Rong. A specific example of how maps shed new light on the interpretation of network data is given in Illustration #1, below. However, presenting graphs of relations using correct locations for villages raises important problems for preserving confidentiality. If we were to present the social networks overlaid on a map of the entire district of Nang Rong with correct village locations and district boundaries indicated on the map, responses to village survey questions could be traced to specific villages. This, in turn, conflicts with the need to maintain confidentiality based on assurances given to respondents in the village survey. There are several ways to guard against a breach of confidentiality. One approach is to alter the map in some way, e.g., by transposing and reorienting it. Another approach, the one we have followed, is to present graphs for sub-regions of the district without specifying their exact location within the district.

The spatial analytic capabilities of the GIS have also been important to our work, allowing us to examine relationships between spatial properties and social network features. We have used the spatial analytic capabilities to measure distances between villages, to locate rivers, perennial streams and bridges between villages, to measure the distance from each village to the district boundary, and to characterize land cover in the territory surrounding each village.

We have calculated and compared the average Euclidean distance traversed by ties between villages on different social network relations. Sharing of elementary schools and temples is more local than renting agricultural equipment and hiring temporary labor, for example. Distance estimates are also important to the consideration of error in the social network data, as illustrated below. Outliers—that is, ties spanning an unusual distance—suggest possible reporting and recording problems in the data. Ties between villages sharing an elementary school are 2.11 km on average and those linking villages sharing a temple are 1.48 km. Whereas, ties based on agricultural equipment and temporary labor are 4.77 and 5.28 km, respectively (Faust et al. 1999, page 326).

Distance to the district boundary allows us to see whether villages in close proximity to the district boundary have more ties to villages outside Nang Rong district than villages far from the district boundary. If so, we might want to re-consider the assumption that the district boundary coincides with the village network boundary. We have found that distance to the district boundary was not correlated with the volume of shared temples and elementary schools, but that villages close to the district boundary had significantly more secondary schools and temporary labor ties to villages outside the district. Surprisingly, villages close to the boundary were less likely to have tractor hiring ties outside the district.

Land cover classifications derived from satellite data were used to consider the association between cropping and the movement of equipment and labor among villages. For example, we have found that the cultivation of upland crops (such as cassava, corn, and sugar cane) coincides with the hiring of large tractors between villages. The greater the percent of a 1.5 km buffer around a village that consists of upland agriculture, the more active the village is in both sending and receiving large tractors.

As in Laumann et al.'s Chapter 1 in this volume, we found that spatial proximity influences network interactions, though the effect of proximity varies by type of relation. Social relations, such as sharing elementary schools and temples, are quite local and are more likely to be disrupted by geographic barriers such as perennial streams and rivers. Economic relations, such as hiring large tractors and movement of labor, cover longer distances and are less likely to be disrupted by geographic barriers. Finally, we found that the presence of a perennial stream between two villages greatly reduces the likelihood of a tie between them, though the effect is somewhat reduced by the presence of a bridge.

7.5 ILLUSTRATIVE FINDINGS

We are still analyzing the social network data from the Nang Rong surveys. So rather than attempt to summarize all the key findings, we present three illustrations from ongoing research. The first shows how the georeferencing of social network data within the GIS has shed new light on the interpretation of the data. The second relates experience from an analysis of contraceptive choice that shows the importance of boundary definition. The third uses comparable social network questions in fifty-one villages to describe variation in patterns of social organization across villages.

7.5.1 Visualization and error

In addition to the GIS results noted above, visualization through the GIS turned out to be of assistance in identifying problems with the lists used to record ties between villages, and with coding based on those lists. Drawing on results reported in Faust et al. (1999), we present two examples, one illustrating problems associated with an incomplete list and the other, problems with duplicate names on the list. In hindsight, it is easy to see how to handle each of these problems, and we have done so in the 2000 round of data collection. We were not aware of them at the time of the 1994/95 data collection, however. Further, we might never have suspected them if we had not incorporated the 1994 community data into the GIS and mapped ties between villages. To provide a clear understanding of the problems, we first describe more specifically the organization and use of village lists in the 1994 community survey, the source of the data for the two examples.

Community data were collected in a group interview of the village headman and other village leaders. Questions were asked about ties to other villages. Interviewers had a list of all the villages in Nang Rong against which they could check and code responses. The list of villages was organized by subdistrict, the administrative units of which districts are composed. There were two problems with this list. First, village names were not unique. There are nineteen instances in which two villages have the same name, eight instances in which three villages share a name, and four instances in which four, five, six, or seven villages have the same name (involving a total of 84 from the 310 villages). Responses to the village network questions often were coded after the interview was complete. Duplicate names could have posed a problem. Interviewers might not know which of a pair or triplet of villages was intended, or may have been unaware or forgotten that a given name might refer to more than one village. Second, the list only included villages, and therefore it omitted other administrative units such as towns where schools or temples could be located.

In our analyses we incorporated the village networks into the GIS using georeferenced village locations. Ties were then displayed as directed arrows between linked villages, with a separate map for each relation. We suspected errors when lines between villages seemed to violate an otherwise orderly pattern. For example, the temple and elementary school networks are generally local, but there are some instances of villages more than ten kilometers apart apparently linked through a shared temple or elementary school. Those ties could be based on kinship relations or prior residences of villagers, but we also wondered about the possibility of data coding error involving duplicate village names. Two pairs of villages more than ten kilometers apart apparently share a temple, and seven pairs of villages more than ten kilometers apart apparently share an elementary school, according to the survey data. For temple sharing, for both pairs, one of the villages involved in the pair has a name duplicated somewhere else in the data set. For elementary schools, this is true for four of the seven pairs of distant villages. Thus, it seems quite likely that duplicate names lie behind coding error. The presence of such suspect ties would not be apparent without taking spatial location into account.

Another kind of data problem could be seen in the spatial patterning of isolates in one of the networks. In the secondary school network, there is a concentration of isolates in the middle of the district. The absence of arrows to and from villages in this region appears to show that these villages do not send children to secondary school. This led us to consider more carefully how data on schools were collected. In the community questionnaire, villagers were asked to name other *villages* to which children went for secondary school. The question format and recording of responses inadvertently omitted the secondary school located in the district *town*, located roughly in the center of the district.

7.5.2 *Open versus closed networks*

This illustration considers the question of whether village position within a network of labor hiring affected women's contraceptive choices. Movements of temporary labor between villages provided potential bridges between otherwise unconnected social groups, and as such, could increase exposure to new information, not only of those who traveled for work but also of others in the home village. We were interested in whether village centrality in networks of labor hiring affected choice of injection, a relatively new method in the Nang Rong context. Our key hypothesis was: The more central the village, the more likely and the earlier that women who live there will hear about and adopt injection. To test this hypothesis, we specified a simplified multilevel model of temporary method choice (pill, IUD, injection, none). Entwisle and Godley (1999) report the findings. Here, we discuss the measurement of village centrality, specifically whether the focus is on ties between villages within Nang Rong or also includes ties beyond the district boundaries, and consequences for the results obtained (Entwisle and Godley 1999).

Information about labor exchange between villages was collected in the community survey:

"Go To"
Q. 69. Sometimes, do villagers in this village go to other villages to work as daily wage laborers?
Q. 70. To which villages do they most often go to work?
"Come From"
Q. 74. Sometimes, does this village require laborers from other villages?
Q. 75. From which villages do they mostly come?

Both sets of questions generate networks of labor exchange between villages. We refer to the first as the "go to" network, and the second as the "come from" network.

Our first approach to the measurement of village position used the complete network of ties within the district. All 310 administratively defined villages in Nang Rong district were part of the village survey in 1994. We organized answers to the labor hiring questions into two 310 × 310 sociomatrices, one for "go to" and the other for "come from." We analyzed these matrices calculating measures of centrality, centralization, and component size and membership. Both networks consisted of a handful of components, which altogether included about 80 percent of the villages. The components in the "go to" network were 236, 10, 2, and 2 in size; the components in the "come from" network were 229, 6, 2, and 2 in size. Only twenty-three of the 310 villages neither sent nor received workers. Labor hiring within Nang Rong district thus linked most of the villages, directly or indirectly. Of interest for the analysis of temporary method choice were measures of degree centrality based on these sociomatrices.

We hypothesized that village centrality within a network of labor hiring would have a positive effect on choice of injection relative to other temporary methods or no method at all. In the multilevel analysis of contraceptive choice, both centrality measures ("go to" and "come from") had significant effects. Surprisingly, one of the measures had a negative rather than a positive effect on injection use. We considered possible reasons why the results failed to confirm our hypothesis: (*a*) village position in a network of temporary labor hiring was poorly measured; (*b*) labor hiring networks were unstable, changing from 1 year to the next; (*c*) these networks form in response to economic factors not controlled in the analysis; (*d*) another set of ties between villages was more relevant to contraceptive choice. We also considered the consequences of ignoring ties to villages outside of the district.

It turns out that villages send ("go to") short-term workers to an average of 3.9 villages: 1.6 villages within Nang Rong district; 1.3 outside the district but in the province; and 1.0 outside the province. All villages are connected to at least one other village in this way—there are no isolates. This interconnectedness may be a feature of modern Nang Rong, coinciding with a greater integration of the region into the national economy. The villages in our sample receive short-term workers from an average of 2.0 other villages: 1.8 within and 0.2 outside the district. Although most hire in workers for temporary help with seasonal agricultural activities, a substantial minority (37 percent) do not. In contrast to the "go to" network, the "come from" network involves fewer and more local ties.

We reanalyzed the data, using counts of ties to other villages, and distinguishing between ties to villages within and outside the district. It turns out that the connection to other villages by virtue of outward short-term labor movements enhanced use of injection, and also of the pill. The number of "go to" ties has a positive and statistically significant effect on both. In contrast, connections to other villages by virtue of the hiring of labor had no effect on temporary method choice. We believe that the contrast between these results shows the importance of ties spanning a long distance. To further confirm this, we disaggregated the "go to" ties, distinguishing between ties to other villages in Nang Rong district, ties to villages outside the district but within Buriram Province, and ties outside the province. Ties to other provinces are especially important for injection use. There are many reasons why use of injection in Nang Rong quadrupled between 1984 and 1994. Nevertheless, our results suggest a role for the diffusion of information (and perhaps the provision of services) along ties defined by the movement of short-term labor. Recently married women are more likely to choose injection if they live in villages central in labor-hiring networks, especially those with ties to villages in other provinces. A more general lesson is that it can be quite misleading to look at network effects within a limited bounded community, a potential problem with the "sociocentric" approach (Laumann et al., Chapter 1, this volume) that studies network ties within a fixed population of actors. Such an approach would likely miss "bridge" actors who link communities and can be critical in disease transmission.

7.5.3 *Variation in household networks across villages*

Replication across settings is an important feature of many of the studies in this volume. The study of Rothenberg et al. (Chapter 5, this volume) contrasts networks in Flagstaff and Atlanta using a methodology developed in the Colorado Springs study (Potterat et al., Chapter 4, this volume). Though focused in Chicago, the CHSLS study by Laumann, Mahay, Paik, and Youm compares patterns of sexual relations between neighborhoods (Laumann and Youm 1999), and the AddHealth study includes multiple high schools. Our final illustration also draws on replicated networks. Having the same network measurement strategy across fifty-one villages allows us to consider whether patterns of social organization are similar or different across villages. An often implicit assumption of network case studies is that a single group or community is representative of other communities or groups. In other words, that results can be generalized to similar settings. However, without replication, this is a critical assumption, which is untested.

In this section, we describe some of the variability among villages in patterns of network ties among households, using two villages and two relations for illustration. We selected these two villages to contrast the patterns and level of ties across households. We also look at two relations, one economic and one kinship. The first relation is help with the rice harvest, and the way this social network was generated was discussed above in Section 7.4.2. The second relation consists of sibling ties between households. For household members aged 18–35 years old, locations of their siblings were recorded. The question asked was:

Q. 4.5. Does this person have other siblings besides the ones [living in the household] that are still living? If they do, record their current location: In this village, in another village in Nang Rong, in another district in Buriram, or in another province.

Figure 7.3 shows the help with the rice harvest networks for two villages. Clearly there are notable differences between these two villages. In village A, households are much more actively involved in helping with the rice harvest than they are in village B. On average, households in village A mentioned receiving help from 2.06 households, as compared with an average of 0.51 mentioned in village B. In Fig. 7.3, the "star" pattern in village A shows that there are a small number of households that are receiving a great deal of help. One household in this village mentioned receiving help from forty-nine other households, and eight mentioned receiving help from more than ten households. In village B the maximum number of households mentioned is five. This difference among households in the amount of help received shows differential centralization of the two villages, as reflected in the variance of the number of households from which help was received. The variances in the number of households from which help was received are 51.18 in village A and 1.10 in village B. Clearly village A is not only more active but also more centralized. This centralization suggests a great deal of variation within the village in the extent to which households are involved in rice cultivation or variation in the amount of land cultivated. We might speculate that this is related to economic or occupational variation in the village.

The pattern of network subgroups also differs between the two villages on this relation. In village B there are eight components ranging in size from two to twenty-five households and involving 57 percent of the households in the village.[8] In village A there is a single component containing 98 percent of the households. There is a clear difference between these two villages in how "connected" households are through rice harvest help ties.

---

[8] A component is a connected subgraph. All actors within a component can be reached via paths of ties between other actors. We report "weak" components. The paths between actors may include ties going in either direction—either to or from the other actors.

(a)

(b)

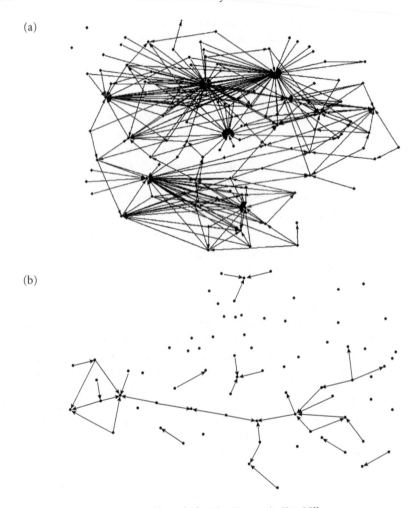

Figure 7.3. *Help with the Rice Harvest in Two Villages*

In comparing these agricultural or economic ties in these two villages, it is important to note that there is considerable variation across Nang Rong district in types of agricultural activity. Some villages are heavily involved in rice cultivation, whereas others cultivate upland crops (cassava, corn, and sugar cane). We might expect that the level of rice harvest help in the villages is related to differences in agricultural activity. We can investigate this using information from the GIS. For each village, a 1.5-km buffer around the village was defined, and the percent of land in rice cultivation, forest, and upland agriculture was calculated (Evans 1998). In village A, 83 percent of the land is in rice cultivation, 8 percent in forest, and the remaining 9 percent in upland agriculture. In contrast, village B has only 52 percent in rice cultivation, 25 percent in forest, and 22 percent in upland agriculture. This pattern is consistent with the different levels of rice harvest help.

(a)

(b)

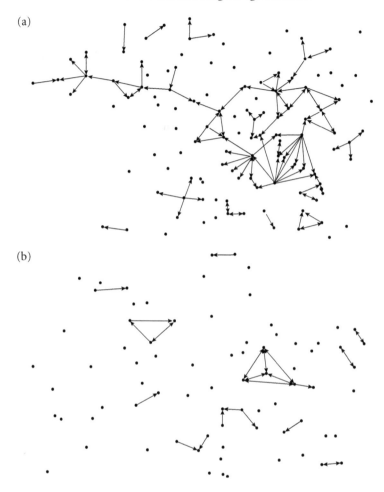

Figure 7.4. *Sibling Ties in Two Villages*

Figure 7.4 shows graphs of the sibling networks. These networks also differ from each other in the two villages, though not as dramatically as help with the rice harvest. The most notable difference between the two villages is a very low level of sibling ties in village B. In this village, 62 percent of households do not have sibling ties to other households in the village; they are "isolates." In village A, 30 percent of households are isolates on the sibling relation. The average number of ties per household also differs between the villages. Households nominated 0.53 other households, on average, in village B and nominated 1.07 in village A. The subgroup patterns also differ. In village B there are eight components, ranging in size from two to five households. In village A there are ten components, ranging in size from two to 57.

Households in village A are more densely tied to one another on both help with the rice harvest and on sibling relationships than is the case in village B. Nevertheless, it is interesting to note that in neither village does rice harvest help go along with sibling ties. In village B there are no instances in which a household nominated another as providing rice harvest help and also as the location of a sibling. In village A there are only eight such instances (0.06 percent of all possible pairs of households). In neither village is it the case that kinship relations, through sibling ties, are the basis for provision of help with the rice harvest. We expect that the links are intergenerational— a hypothesis that we plan to investigate with more recent data.

In sum, only with social networks measured comparably across settings can we investigate the extent of variability in network patterns. In the example described here there are large differences, especially in networks of economic cooperation. In our ongoing work, we are investigating this variability across all fifty-one villages, and to study how variation in network patterns is related to other characteristics of the villages, such as agricultural activity and village history.

7.6 SOCIAL NETWORK DATA IN THE 2000/2001 SURVEYS

By way of conclusion we discuss the social network components of the 2000 round of data collection, which incorporated changes in life styles in Nang Rong, changes in technology that can be used in data gathering, and changes in administrative infrastructure in Nang Rong. We capture more aspects of interaction opportunities in Nang Rong villages and we take advantage of developments since the 1994 round of data collection. In so doing, we opted to retain as many of the social network components as possible from the 1994 round in order to look at change over time. In some cases this is likely to mean that some of the relations will be sparser than in 1994 because of ongoing changes in the villages. For example, anecdotal evidence suggests that as the economy continues to move from subsistence to market the role of local rice mills as a gathering place has changed. Increasingly, villagers are selling their rice harvest to merchants who then take the rice out of the village to be milled at larger, more efficient mills. Villagers then buy the rice they consume at stores. We have decided to keep the rice mill questions to see if the anecdotal evidence is correct, to be able to document how social change affects the nature of social interaction, and to see who the leaders and laggards are.

Three new social network generators are based on propinquity and advances in our ability to measure it. Since our last round of data collection, it has become easier to measure geographic location and include this information in a Geographic Information System. We use official records to obtain the locations and names of owners for all land in Nang Rong that has been recorded in one of the two agencies charged with overseeing land claims and ownership. The locations were digitized into a GIS, along with ID numbers unique to each plot. The list of names of owners, along with the same unique plot specific ID numbers will be merged, by name,[9]

---

[9] There are a number of reasons why Thai names are much more likely to be unique than American, European, Korean, or Chinese names. Put differently, in Thailand the John Smith problem is less likely to arise. Surnames were not used in Thailand until King Rama VI decreed that they should be used. This decree came out about 1920, and thus family names have only been used for a few generations.

with data collected in the household interviews. This procedure provides adjacencies of land owned by villagers. Once we have this, a wide variety of social network measures can be constructed. For example, for any given pair of households that owns land, we can measure the number of parcels that lie between them (or the distance or travel time between them), as well as whether their parcels are adjacent. We can also see how these adjacencies intersect other relations, such as kinship or help with the rice harvest.

While owners of adjacent properties are likely to interact with one another, users of adjacent properties are even more likely to interact as they go through the normal routines of planting, weeding, and harvesting crops. This is particularly likely in Nang Rong where plots tend to be small, there is relatively little mechanization of agricultural tasks, and the planting of most plots is tied to the timing of the annual monsoon.

We are using the social networks that exist in Nang Rong to measure plot use adjacencies. At the community level, we ask knowledgeable informants where households in the village are farming. The emphasis is on use and not ownership. Using maps that have aerial photographs as background, these knowledgeable individuals draw the outlines of plots used by villagers, and put in each plot a running ID number. While they are drawing these plot lines, we also maintain a list with the same running numbers and the names of the household heads that use the plots. If there is an adjacent plot that is used by someone from some other village, their name and village number is recorded. Then during the household interview, respondents are asked about the agricultural plots that they use, including the names and village numbers of their neighbors for the four cardinal directions. Households know their farming neighbors and there are knowledgeable individuals within a village who can draw the plot lines while providing us with the names of those who use those plots.[10] By matching, we are able to link households to the plots

Further, when families were registering their surnames, there were checks to make sure that there were no duplicates. Thus in principle in the 1920s each family had a unique surname. While the checking for duplicates at registration time was by hand, and hence not perfect, the overall effect was to have the vast majority of surnames be unique. Today, if you want to change your surname, you have to go to the registrar's office and they will check to see if your proposed new surname duplicates the surname of anyone else in the country. If it is a duplicate, they have to pick another one.

Unlike many Western countries, there is no tendency for fathers to give their first names to their son or mothers to give their first name to their daughter. Instead, sometimes a syllable from the mother's name and a syllable from the father's name might be joined to create a name for the child. In short, frequently first names are made up, and thus have a higher probability of being unique.

The Thai alphabet has forty-four consonants, twenty-one vowels and five intonations. Hence, there is a greater possibility for creating a wide range of unique names than in the Western alphabet.

A computerized file exists containing the names of approximately 40,000 individuals who were listed in the household rosters of the 1994 data collection. In this file, there were only 130 cases where more that one person had the same first and last name.

[10] Village headmen, assistant headmen, and village committee members tend to know where people in the village farm. In addition, in recent work in rice growing areas, we have found that hunters are also a reliable source of information. These are individuals who hunt for frogs, field rats, or crabs. In order to hunt on someone's field, they need their permission, and hence they know who uses which fields. The same is the case for those who fish in the rice growing areas during the times when they are flooded.

they use, and do so both within our GIS and in our regular SAS data management file. (This procedure is discussed in considerable detail in Rindfuss et al.
2003) Again, we can construct a variety of social network measures from this
data, including whether pairs of households use adjacent plots, the distances
between the plots they use, and the number of other plots intermediate between
their plots.

The third propinquity measure involves obtaining the location of all dwelling
units within our study villages. The social network argument is that households that
are physically closer to one another will be more likely to interact. Since the 1994
round of data collection, the GPS became fully operational. This is a system of
twenty-four satellites that orbit the earth. With a handheld GPS device, as long as one
can read at least three of these satellites, one can obtain a reading from the GPS
device that indicates the present location, and which, in turn, can be corrected for the
error that is in the GPS and then incorporated into an existing GIS. Once the data are
in the GIS, a wide variety of social network measures can be calculated.

We also obtain the name of the school attended by all household members. Both
primary and secondary schools have names that are unique within the district. The
idea is to be able to determine who within the village were classmates, on the assumption that classmates will be more likely to interact with one another. In addition,
since many primary and secondary schools have catchments that span more than one
village, the social networks formed in school will likely link across villages. After they
leave school these ties get reinforced when they see each other at fairs, markets, and
so forth. Over time, the catchments for secondary schools have become smaller as
more secondary schools are built, and hence the geographic areas networked will
decrease.

Finally, while not strictly a social network variable, we collect information about
the dwelling unit where households live with an eye toward the architecture, whether
it is likely to facilitate or hinder social interactions with non-household members. A
traditional dwelling unit in this part of Thailand was made of wood resting on pil-
ings that raised the structure approximately one story above ground level. See panel
A of Fig. 7.5. The ground level was typically open, sometimes with a secure area to
keep animals at night. Cooking was done outside, underneath the house. Given the
tropical climate, a substantial amount of living and socializing took place in the
shade underneath the house. Examples of activities that would have typically
occurred under the house include food preparation, silk weaving, and basket making. Houses are clustered close together within villages, and with many daily activities occurring outdoors, underneath the house, conversations with neighbors can
happen easily.

As Nang Rong becomes more affluent, housing styles are changing. One of the
first steps is to enclose part of the area underneath the house, and this becomes the
kitchen (panel B of Fig. 7.5). Then at some stage the entire area underneath the
house is enclosed, typically using cinder block (panel C of Fig. 7.5). At this point,
more of everyday life is taking place within the confines of the dwelling unit. Unless
there is a porch or some other outdoor gathering place, the type of casual conversations that used to take place become less likely. Further, some dwelling units now

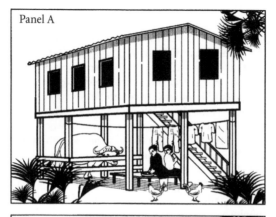

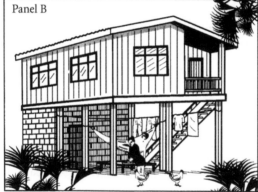

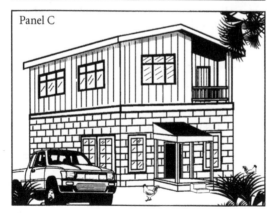

Figure 7.5. *Examples of Nang Rong Housing Styles*

have an air conditioner, likely making the household turn more inward. We measured these variables. Given that the richer families are the ones that first fill in the area under the house, this may lead to divisions between the rich and those who are not so rich.

References

Borgatti, S., Everett, M. et al. (1999). *UCINET 5.0 Version 1.00 for Windows: Software for Social Network Analysis.* Harvard, MA: Natick Analytic Technologies.

Boyd, M. (1989). "Family and personal networks in international migration: Recent developments and new agendas," *International Migration Review*, 23(3): 638–70.

Chung, W. (1993). "The diffusion of fertility control in Korea: Multilevel models for social network data." PhD Dissertation, State University of New York at Stony Brook.

Clarke, K. (1990). *Analytical and Computer Cartography.* Englewood Cliffs, NJ: Prentice Hall.

Entwisle, B. and Godley, J. (1999). "Village networks and patterns of contraceptive choice in Nang Rong, Thailand." Unpublished manuscript.

—— Rindfuss, R. R. et al. (1996). "Community and contraceptive choice in rural Thailand: A case study of Nang Rong," *Demography*, 33: 1–11.

Evans, Tom, P. (1998). "Integration of community-level social and environmental data: Spatial modeling of community boundaries in northeast Thailand." PhD Dissertation, Department of Geography, University of North Carolina at Chapel Hill.

Faust, K., Entwisle, B. et al. (1999). "Spatial arrangement of social and economic networks among villages in Nang Rong district, Thailand," *Soc Nets*, 21: 311–337.

Fukui, H. (1993). *Food and Population in a Northeast Thai Village. Monographs of the Center for Southeast Asian Studies.* Honolulu, University of Hawaii Press.

Jato, M., van der Straten, A. et al. (1995). "Women's 'Tontines' in Yaounde, Cameroon: Using social networks for family planning communication." The Johns Hopkins School of Public Health, Project Report No. 6.

Kincaid, D., Massiah, E. et al. (1993). Communication networks, ideation, and family planning in Trishal, Bangladesh." Paper presented at the annual meetings of the Population Association of America, Cincinatti, OH.

Kohler, H.-P. (1997). "Fertility and social interaction: An economic approach." PhD Dissertation, University of California at Berkeley.

Laumann, E. and Youm, Y. (1999). "Racial/ethnic group differences in the prevalence of sexually transmitted diseases in the United States: A network explanation," *Sex Transm Dis*, 26: 250–61.

Massey, D. S., Alarcon, R. et al. (1987). *Return to Aztlan: The Social Process of International Migration from Western Mexico.* Berkeley, CA: University of California Press.

Mita, R. and Simmons, R. (1995). "Diffusion of the culture of contraception: Program effects on young women in rural Bangladesh," *Stud Fam Plann*, 26: 1–13.

Montgomery, M. R. and Casterline, J. B. (1993). "The diffusion of fertility control in Taiwan: Evidence from pooled cross-section time-series models," *Population Stud*, 47: 457–76.

National Statistics Office (1990). Population and housing census. Changwat, Buriram, Thailand: Office of the Prime Minister.

Parnwell, M. J. G. (1988). "Rural poverty, development, and the environment: The case of North-East Thailand," *J Biogeo*, 15: 199–213.

Rigg, J. (1991). "Homogeneity and heterogeneity: An analysis of the nature of variation in Northeastern Thailand," *Malaysian J Tropical Geography*, 22: 63–72.

Rindfuss, R., Kaneda, T. et al. (2003). "Panel studies and migration," under review.

Rindfuss, R. R., Prasartkul, P. et al. (2003). "Household—parcel linkages in Nang Rong, Thailand: Challenges of large samples." In Jefferson Fox, Ronald R. Rindfuss, S. J. Walsh, and V. Mishra (eds.), *People and the Environment: Approaches for Linking Household and Community Surveys to Remote Sensing and GIS.* Boston MA: Kluwer Academic Publishers, pp. 131–72.

Valente, T. W. (1995). *Network Models of the Diffusion of Innovations.* New Jersey: Hampton Press.

Watkins, Susan Cotts (1991). *From Provinces in to Nations: Demographic Integration in Western Europe, 1870–1960.* Princeton, NJ: Princeton University Press.

8

Social and Sexual Networks: The National Longitudinal Study of Adolescent Health

PETER S. BEARMAN, JAMES MOODY,
KATHERINE STOVEL, AND LISA THALJI

8.1 INTRODUCTION

The predominant threats to adolescents' health and well-being stem from the choices that adolescents make and the behaviors they engage in. For example, becoming pregnant, acquiring a sexually transmitted disease (STD), suffering a violent accident, considering suicide, beginning to smoke, and developing a weight problem are all at least in part attributable to behaviors and choices that adolescents make in conjunction with others around them (Bauman and Fisher 1986; Smith and Crawford 1986; Hayes 1987; Adcock et al. 1991; Bearman 1991; Jeanneret 1992; Thompson 1995; Resnick et al. 1997). Therefore, to systematically study the determinants of the health of adolescents, research must focus on a complex constellation of factors that influence adolescent behavior. The most fundamental of these are the social contexts and relationships in which adolescents are embedded. With this in mind, the National Longitudinal Study of Adolescent Health (hereafter, *Add Health*) was explicitly designed to provide

The material in this chapter was presented at the International Union for the Scientific Study of Population (IUSSP) Committee on AIDS Conference on Partnership Networks and the Spread of HIV and Other Infections, Chiang Mai, Thailand, February 2000. This research is based on data from the *Add Health* project, a program project designed by J. Richard Udry (PI) and Peter Bearman, and funded by grant P01-HD31921 from the National Institute of Child Health and Human Development to the Carolina Population Center, University of North Carolina at Chapel Hill, with cooperative funding participation by the National Cancer Institute; the National Institute of Alcohol Abuse and Alcoholism; the National Institute on Deafness and Other Communication Disorders; the National Institute on Drug Abuse; the National Institute of General Medical Sciences; the National Institute of Mental Health; the National Institute of Nursing Research; the Office of AIDS Research, National Institute of Health (NIH); the Office of Behavior and Social Science Research, NIH; the Office of the Director, NIH; the Office of Research on Women's Health, NIH; the Office of Population Affairs, DHHS; the National Center for Health Statistics, Centers for Disease Control and Prevention, DHHS; the Office of Minority Health, Centers for Disease Control and Prevention, DHHS; the Office of Minority Health, Office of Public Health and Science, DHHS; the Office of the Assistant Secretary for Planning and Evaluation, DHHS; and the National Science Foundation. Persons interested in obtaining data files from The National Longitudinal Study of Adolescent Health should contact *Add Health*, Carolina Population Center, 123 West Franklin Street, Chapel Hill, NC 27516-3997 (email: addhealth@unc.edu).

detailed measurement from a large nationally representative sample on the most central social contexts and relationships that influence the health status of adolescents. The specific contexts focused in *Add Health* are: families, dyadic friendships, peer groups, romantic and sexual partners, schools, neighborhoods, and communities (Resnick et al. 1997).

As is described in greater detail below, the highly clustered community-based design of *Add Health* is unusual, but one of its primary benefits is that it provides information from multiple sources from which we can generate images of the social and relational world of adolescents. In addition to collecting extensive self-report and network data from over 90,000 adolescents in eighty communities, *Add Health* collected data on family relations from parents and siblings; on the composition of peer groups from adolescents' friends; on romantic relationships from romantic partners; on geographic proximity from global positioning system (GPS) data; and on schools from other students and school administrators. As a result, *Add Health* provides measurement of multiple levels of context from multiple perspectives, making it possible to interweave spatial and social networks and to construct models of health risk based on real patterns of association within the adolescent world.

We begin this chapter by outlining the major design features of the *Add Health* study, the sample structure, and the fieldwork experience. We then describe how social and sexual networks are measured in *Add Health*, and discuss some studies that illustrate the type of analyses that are possible with these data. We conclude with a brief overview of the network design elements proposed for the next wave of *Add Health* data collection.

8.2 DESIGN OVERVIEW OF *ADD HEALTH*

Concern with the collection of linked social and sexual network data is reflected in the unusual design of the *Add Health* study.[1] Rather than sample adolescents randomly from the population at large, *Add Health* rests on a multistage, clustered sampling design. At the first stage, we drew a nationally representative sample of high schools ($n = 80$), and enrolled all students attending each sampled school; from these students we selected a representative sample of adolescents for further in-depth study. Between 1994 and 1996, *Add Health* collected three waves of data: the initial school-based survey, the in-depth in-home interview of a subset of students identified in the school-based study (*Wave I*; $n = 20{,}745$) and a follow-up in-home interview approximately 1 year later (*Wave II*; $n = 14{,}738$).[2] Parents of adolescents who participated in the in-home phases of the study were also asked to complete a questionnaire, and school administrators completed a brief questionnaire in the first and third years of the study. Ultimately producing a nationally representative study of American adolescents in grades 7–12, this design allowed us to collect—for the first

---

[1] Additional details about the study design can be found in (Bearman et al. 1996).

[2] We did not follow respondents who were high school seniors at *Wave I*, so our loss to follow-up was not actually as severe as it appears from the difference in *n*'s between *Wave I* and *Wave II*.

time ever—complete social network data describing the structure of adolescent relationships in many different American communities.

8.2.1 Sample details and design features

The primary sampling frame for *Add Health* was derived from the Quality Education Database, which lists all high schools in the United States. Schools were stratified by region, urbanicity, school type (public, private, parochial), ethnic mix, and size; the *Add Health* sample of schools consists of eighty high schools (defined as schools with an eleventh grade and more than thirty students) selected from this list with probability proportional to size. For each sampled high school, *Add Health* identified and recruited one of its feeder schools (typically a middle school) with probability proportional to its student contribution to the high school. Almost 70 percent of the contacted schools agreed to participate in the study, however for schools that refused, *Add Health* replaced them with another school (or school-pair) selected from the same strata. The final sample of schools consists of school pairs from eighty different communities, and includes private, religious, and public schools from communities located in urban, suburban, and rural areas of the country.[3] All students attending one of the sampled schools were asked to complete the in-school questionnaire, which contained basic social and demographic information, as well as an extensive social network module (described below).

Between September 1994 and April 1995, the paper and pencil, op-scan in-school questionnaire was administered to all students in each sampled school. Each school administration occurred on a single day within one 45–60 min class period, and we made no effort to include students not in school on the day of the administration. Nevertheless, over 80 percent of the enrolled students completed the questionnaire. Though seven of our recruited schools ultimately did not allow us to survey students in the school (but did provide us with a roster for subsequent sampling purposes) we have in-school questionnaire data from 90,118 students attending 141 schools.

Sampling for the second stage of data collection (the *Wave I* in-home survey) proceeded from the population of students identified in the in-school phase. From the union of students on school rosters and students not on a roster who completed an in-school questionnaire, *Add Health* randomly selected 200 students from each community and administered a 90-min computer assisted (CASI) in-home interview. Since students who did not complete the in-school survey but were on a sampled school's roster were eligible to be selected for participation in the in-home main sample, the *Wave I* sample includes students who had dropped out of school. Numerous supplementary special samples were drawn and adolescents in these groups were interviewed as well. *Add Health* completed 20,745 *Wave I* in-home interviews, with an 80 percent response rate. Parental interviews are available for slightly more than 85 percent of all adolescents in the in-home sample.

---

[3] Because some sampled high schools included a middle school, the actual number of schools included in the study is 141.

In two large and twelve small schools, we attempted in-home and parent interviews for *all* students enrolled in a high school or middle school. The two large high
schools were selected purposefully: one is a predominantly White school located in a
small town ($n \approx 1000$ students); the other is characterized by substantial ethnic
heterogeneity and is located in a major metropolitan area ($n \approx 1700$ students). The
twelve smaller schools are located in rural and urban areas; both public and private
schools are represented ($n \approx 150$ students per school). Because we surveyed all students in these schools, they generate a large number of romantic and friendship pairs
in which both members of the pair completed the in-depth in-home interviews.
Therefore, for these schools we have much more complete images of the social
networks and romantic partnerships in which adolescents are embedded.

Approximately 1 year after the *Wave I* interview, we conducted follow-up interviews with most of the adolescents who participated in the first wave of the in-home
survey. Follow-up interviews were not attempted with *Wave I* seniors at *Wave II*. Over
88 percent of all eligible *Wave I* respondents participated in *Wave II*, resulting in
14,738 interviews.

8.2.2 Design issues and the collection of network data

In addition to serving as the sampling frame for the in-home survey, the in-school
questionnaire is the primary source for complete friendship network data. From a
roster of all students at their school, every student was asked to nominate his or her
five best male and female friends, and to report on whether they had specific types of
contact with each nominated friend. Figure 8.1 reproduces a page of the in-school
questionnaire that was used to collect social network data. Because all students in the
school are surveyed, we have data on the complete school-based friendship network
of adolescents. In addition to the network data, all students were asked to provide
basic social and demographic information, including reporting on their parents'
educational and occupational background, their family's household structure, the
sports and extracurricular activities that they participated in during the school year,
risk-behaviors they engaged in, their visions for the future, their self-esteem, and
their general health status.

Data collected during the in-home phase of *Add Health* provide more detailed
measurement on a much broader range of health-related behaviors and experiences,
including drug and alcohol use, sexual behavior, and criminal activities. Other items
assess overall health status, health utilization, decision-making, family dynamics,
aspirations, and attitudes. Portions of the in-school social network module were
repeated at *Wave I*, though since not *all* students complete this phase it is not possible to generate complete models of network position (except in the saturated settings).[4] Nevertheless, this data provides rich ego-based network information. Most
importantly for those interested in the spread of infections, in addition to collecting

---

[4] The laptops used to collect data at *Wave I* were each loaded with the Student Directory information
for each school so that adolescents to nominate their friends and partners.

The next questions are about your female friends. First list their names on the line marked "Name." Then, just as you did for other household members and for male friends, look them up in the Student Directory and write their student numbers in the boxes below their names. Then, darken the ovals that correspond to the student numbers.

Look back at the EXAMPLE on page 6 if you need help with this. If a friend goes to a school for which you don't have a directory, give her the number 7777. (If your friend isn't in school at all, give her the number 7777 also.) If your friend goes to your school and isn't listed in the Student Directory, give her the number 9999; if your friend goes to the other school and isn't listed, give her the number 8888.

Remember: If a female friend goes to your school but is not listed in the directory, write 9999.
　　　　　 If a female friend goes to the other school but is not listed in the directory, write 8888.
　　　　　 If a female friend does not go to your school or the other school, write 7777.

After you have listed your female friends and their numbers, answer the five questions about each of them.

YOUR FEMALE FRIENDS

List your closest female friends. List your best female friend first, then your next best friend,
and so on. Boys may include girls who are friends and girlfriends.

	Best Female Friend 1	Female Friend 2	Female Friend 3	Female Friend 4	Female Friend 5
Name:					
Number:					

Darken the oval under the name if:

39. you went to her house in the
last seven days......①......②......③......④......⑤

40. you met her after school to
hang out or go somewhere
in the last seven days......①......②......③......④......⑤

41. you spent time with her last
weekend......①......②......③......④......⑤

42. you talked with her about a
problem in the last seven days......①......②......③......④......⑤

43. you talked with her on the
telephone in the last seven days......①......②......③......④......⑤

Figure 8.1. *Friendship Nomination Page from* Add Health *In-school Survey*

friendship nominations, the *Wave I* instrument collects detailed data on romantic and sexual partnerships during the past 18 months: each adolescent in the in-home sample was asked to nominate up to three recent romantic and three non-romantic sexual partners from the school-based rosters. Even if the nominated partner was not in the in-home sample, we are able to link the nomination to the partners' in-school data, thereby augmenting the data provided by the in-home subject with partners' self-report data.

8.2.3 *Data security*

Because of the clustered design, it is a potentially trivial problem to deductively identify individual data collected for *Add Health*. To reduce the likelihood of any sort of breach of confidentiality, we developed an elaborate and rigorous security system to protect the identities of participating schools and students. The basic principle of the security system is the separation of identities and responses, which we accomplished through a complex identification scheme whereby each respondent was assigned up to five separate identifiers. We subcontracted with York University in Canada to act as the Security Manager and the depository for all identifying information.[5]

8.3 FIELDWORK EXPERIENCE

Fieldwork for the in-school survey and *Waves I* and *II* was conducted by the National Opinion Research Center (NORC). Due to both the massive scale and the clustered design, the fieldwork required to complete *Add Health* was truly unprecedented: the initial goal was to survey almost 100,000 adolescents in 160 schools in eighty communities nation-wide in a year's time. The reality was an aggressive timeline for recruitment of schools and survey administration, constant efforts to prevent negative publicity and community backlash, struggles to conform to the requirements of the security system, and nagging worries that the survey would be canceled midstream.

8.3.1 *In-school component*

Once the sample of schools was drawn, NORC began to recruit schools. This meant sending advance packets of information (advance letters and brochures describing the study) to each sampled school, and then contacting school principals and districts by telephone. However, each school came with its own unique personality and set of procedures. In many instances we encountered reluctance or resistance: for some districts we were required to submit a detailed research proposal, while in others our efforts got caught in bureaucratic swamps. Negotiations were painstakingly lengthy (in some cases as long as 3 months) and at several points senior project staff at NORC or study investigators from the Carolina Population Center got involved in the recruitment efforts.

To counter schools' reluctance to participate, NORC sent specialized letters, followed up with telephone calls, and occasionally arranged for in-person visits by field

---

[5] Throughout the fieldwork, York retained the links between the identifying information and the questionnaire data; NORC retained only the questionnaire data.

staff and senior project staff from NORC and, in some instances, visits by senior study investigators. As a timesavings strategy, we began parallel recruitment efforts in certain strata, though in several cases school visits by the study investigators effectively converted initial refusals into agreements to participate. Our most effective negotiations focused on the benefits the school would enjoy as a result of their participation, as well as on ways to reduce perceived burden to the school. For example, we promised to provide data to the school that would allow them to comparatively assess their students' health, we offered to collect the data over several days, and we offered administrative help with pre-data collection tasks. In addition to negotiating the reduction of burden, we also had to concede to some other special requests, including designing and administering a separate questionnaire for one school and presenting the findings to the entire student body. In other cases, we agreed to limit the number of times we would contact households for the in-home survey. As a last resort, we settled for only a school enrollment roster from which we could draw our in-home sample. We found that the commitment to provide data to schools was a strong incentive to schools, significantly more important than the token financial incentive we were able to provide.

Despite our best efforts, approximately 20 percent of our initially sampled schools refused to participate. Refusals occurred at every step along the way: they occurred prior to agreeing to participate, at the beginning of the school year, immediately before the survey session, and on a couple of occasions on the day of the administration itself. Often the refusals were a result of idiosyncratic factors that could not be anticipated, including an affair between a principal and teacher, an angry parent heavily connected to an active PTA organization, and an upcoming school board election. The top three reasons for school refusals were (*a*) potential backlash from communities and fear of parent organizations' negative mobilization given the linkage between the in-school and the more sensitive in-home survey; (*b*) time away from class instruction; and (*c*) burden on school personnel.

While recruitment efforts continued, we began administering the in-school survey in the fall of 1994. When they agreed to participate in the study, each school had agreed to provide us with a roster of the names of all enrolled students. Though we explicitly requested electronic rosters, and even provided each school with a template, we received roster data in over 100 different formats (and mainly in hardcopy!). As a result, preadministration roster processing was a major undertaking. We keyed and processed the roster data (containing over 100,000 names in total), assigned a special identifier to each student as part of the security system, sorted by girls and boys, and by grade, and produced a Student Directory for each school. We printed tens of thousands of directories, which were used by the students to nominate household member and friends during the survey.

Once a school had agreed to participate in the study, we began the consent process. To comply with federal legislation, we sent special requests for permission to parents of public school children to have their child's name appear in the Student Directory. This special consent to release directory information came on top of our parental permission requirement for the in-school survey.[6] All told, we sent 160,000 times two permission forms out into the universe: we sent one set to schools for the adolescents to carry home, and mailed another set directly to the parents. To placate parents' fears, we established a toll free number and encouraged parents to call with questions or concerns. Parents used this number so much that NORC had to hire a full-time person to answer the toll free line 5 days a week, routing the problem parents to senior staff attention.

Because the schools were asked to host and proctor the survey sessions, it was important that we implemented standardized procedures across all of the sampled schools. We developed In-School Administration Manuals for field staff to train the teachers and proctors on the distribution and secured return of materials. In some instances, despite our requests, schools declined our offer to train their staff. For those schools all we could do was stress the importance of each teacher reading the manual and contacting either the school coordinator or NORC with questions.

The logistical coordination for the preparation and shipment of survey materials to schools was another massive undertaking. We ordered tens of thousands of pencils, preprinted envelopes, questionnaires, boxes, and labels. We prepared specialized "teacher boxes" with all of the survey materials required for each classroom. We mailed the boxes 3 days prior to the Survey Day session using overnight shippers so that boxes could be easily tracked. Even so, schools signed for boxes and subsequently lost them within their own schools. A few school janitors misplaced boxes, others inadvertently threw them out, and yet others were lost by the shippers.

On the days of the administration, we requested that schools issue PA announcements to remind teachers and students of the survey. Field staff and their clerical assistants arrived an hour before the sessions to facilitate the administration and help with any last minute details. At the end of the administration, and in keeping with the security system, students were asked to tear off the first page of the questionnaire (which contained their identifying information) and place it into a special envelope called "names." Next, they placed the questionnaire in another envelope called "answers," and finally, they placed the Student Directory into a third envelope. Teachers placed the permission forms in a fourth envelope.

All materials were returned to a central location where field staff and their clerical assistants carefully checked each and every envelope to ensure the proper contents of each. They then shipped the materials to three separate locations with the first page identifying information shipped to York University, questionnaires to the optical scanning subcontractor, and Student Directories to NORC for shredding.

---

[6] Careful negotiations between NICHD (the federal funding agency) and the Office of Protection from Research Risks, allowed us to use passive parental consent except in those schools or districts that mandated active consent. We feared that requiring active consent forms for participation in the in-school survey would have effectively killed the study. In the end, seven schools required active consent. To bolster the return rate in these schools we helped organize pizza parties to the homerooms that returned the most forms. These tricks did not work. In these schools we also sent home a third set of permission forms. As expected, the final participation rates for these schools was low, ranging from 20–60%.

While most survey sessions were executed without a hitch, we did have our share of excitement. Parents in several communities organized picketing and rallies against the study, and a few principals got cold feet and attempted to cancel the session. But aside from these isolated setbacks, it was a heroic effort on the part of schools and teachers to pull it all off. The excitement in the schools on Survey Days was truly incredible. The students knew something important was happening to them, and to their schools.

8.3.2 *In-home component,* Wave I

In spite of the large number of respondents in the in-school phase of *Add Health*, *Wave I* of the in-home component was the largest field effort NORC had ever undertaken (As originally drawn, the in-home sample consisted of approximately 27,000 adolescents). To mount this portion of the study, NORC hired a huge field force, including 5 field task leaders, 35 field managers, and 511 field interviewers. Because of *Add Health*'s community-based design, we sought to recruit and hire the field interviewers locally.[7] Since approximately 70 percent of our field force had no experience as professional interviewers, we developed a 1-day general training on basic interviewing skills and then a separate 5-day project specific training session, which we held at five separate locations around the country.

We also spent a significant amount of time planning and brainstorming on how to counter and be prepared for (*a*) community backlash; (*b*) diffusion among students; (*c*) organized diffusion among parents to block the survey in their communities; and (*d*) refusals by parents or students to participate in the in-home survey.

The in-home interview had its own set of major logistical coordination issues. We prepared bulk supply boxes for each of the 511 interviewers that included the permission forms, assignment logs, show cards, GPS devices, batteries, and other materials required for the interview. We carefully loaded the questionnaire program and enrollment rosters on 550 laptops and conducted extensive testing before shipment to the interviewers.

As had been the case in the in-school phase, the security system again affected all of the technical and operational procedures, including (*a*) what we could and could not print on field materials; (*b*) our laptop systems and programs (where we incorporated three levels of password protection and double encrypted all software and data); and (*c*) the complicated data transmission protocols that decoupled the identifying information from the actual questionnaire data and transmitted the separate types of files to York University and NORC, respectively.

Data collection began in May 1995 and continued through December 1995, with the majority of the cases completed by September of 1995. Advance letters were mailed to each parent alerting them that an interviewer would visit their home and seeking the parent's consent. Interviewers then knocked on doors to secure consent

---

[7] Though we did not allow any interviewers to work in the neighborhood or community in which they resided, in order to maintain confidentiality.

in person. Both the advance letter and the consent forms again contained a toll free number that parents could call if they had questions or concerns.[8] This time around most parents who called simply wanted to confirm the legitimacy of the survey, though some parents called to refuse.

Across all communities, refusals to the in-home survey were not as much of a problem as we had anticipated; after all of our conversion attempts we had an 80 percent participation rate. Parents and adolescents refused for many of the same reasons that they refuse many health-related surveys: they said they were too busy, they were not interested, they had concerns over privacy, and they felt the subject matter was too sensitive. As far as we could determine, the network components of the study did not factor into the refusal rate.

The adolescent in-home interview was conducted using a computer assisted personal interview (CAPI), and for all sensitive health-status and health-risk behavior questions, (including nomination of romantic and sexual partners) audio-CASI (ACASI) technology.[9] For the CAPI portions of the interview (about two-thirds of the interview), an interviewer asked the adolescent questions and entered the response into a computer; in the ACASI portion, adolescents listened to recordings of questions through earphones and directly keyed their responses into a laptop computer. Before the ACASI portion began, the interviewer turned the laptop around so that the adolescent could view the screen, and trained the adolescent on how to record answers for the self-administered portion.[10]

Most interviews were conducted in the adolescents' homes, but interviews were also administered in backyards, on porches, and even in a McDonalds. The average interview lasted about 90 min. For parents who wanted to see the questionnaire, we included an option in the laptop for them to walk through a blank questionnaire. For parents who wanted to listen to the interview, we gently explained the importance of privacy and standardization. In some instances, parents insisted; when this occurred we did not conduct an interview in that household.

All in all, we found that adolescents really enjoyed completing the interview. In communities where we sampled only 200 adolescents, interviewers were frequently approached by adolescents not selected for the survey and asked if they could participate and why they were not chosen. One feature the adolescents were particularly enthusiastic about was the computer administration. In fact, some adolescents were so adept at using the computer that they continued past the ACASI section and self-administered the last sections, which should have been interviewer-administered.[11]

---

[8] We retained our full-time person who continued to answer calls 5 days per week for the duration of the field period.

[9] ACASI technology has been shown to reduce response bias associated with sensitive questions and nonnormative behavioral items (Turner et al. 1998). We adopted it here in order to reduce the impact of interviewer or parental effects on adolescents' responses to questions about their sexual behavior.

[10] Immediately before the ACASI section the adolescent was given a few practice items so they could develop a sense of the look and feel of the technology.

[11] Once we discovered this was occurring with some regularity, we inserted another password at the end of the ACASI section so that the adolescents could no longer continue on their own.

We also encountered our share of resistance, though most of this was directed toward the schools. In one community, we decided to suspend all further recruitment and interview efforts when a group of parents aggressively mobilized against the study, and in a few other communities we had to temporarily suspend interviewing.

8.3.3 *In-home component,* Wave II

In the spring of 1996, we recontacted approximately 17,000 households.[12] Like *Wave I*, the *Wave II* questionnaire was a 90-min CAPI/ACASI interview that included the school enrollment rosters. Because of the smaller sample, we reduced our field staff for *Wave II*: the field force this time around consisted of 4 task leaders, 24 field managers, and 335 field interviewers. The training program was retooled to take into account what we learned from *Wave I* as well as the new features included for *Wave II*.

The reception we received for *Wave II* was remarkably different from what we encountered at *Wave I*. Now adolescents knew what to expect, and often wanted to participate; this was reflected in our follow-up response rates, which were approximately 90 percent. Parents also seemed more relaxed, and we encountered less negative diffusion and fewer attempts to block the survey from the communities. Wherever possible, we sent the same interviewer who completed the interview in *Wave I* to the *Wave II* household. When this was not possible, some adolescents would say, "Hey, you're not the same lady who was here last year!" At the end, we discovered that we were able to weather the political landmines and logistical challenges posed by the survey design to successfully complete *Add Health*.

8.3.4 *Measurement of network data in* Add Health

Recall that a primary aim of the *Add Health* study was to carefully measure the major social contexts affecting the health and well-being of adolescents. Like many other recent health-related studies (Laumann et al. 1994) *Add Health* collected extensive ego-centered network data. However, because of its unique clustered design (coupled with the fact that adolescents' social worlds tend to be focused on their schools), *Add Health* also was able to collect complete social network data for eighty American communities. Because the *Add Health* study collected friendship nominations from all students who attended each participating school, both individual (ego-) and school-level networks could be constructed. This unique design enables us to comprehensively measure the structure of the extended friendship network each respondent is embedded in, as well as to describe the overall social structure of the respondent's particular school.

In addition to the extensive friendship data collected in the in-school survey, *Add Health* collected two additional waves of friendship nominations, again soliciting opposite sex and same sex friendship nominations from the School Directory. Further, all in-home respondents identified (from the School Directory) up to three

---

[12] As noted above, *Wave I* seniors were not recontacted at *Wave II*.

others with whom they had had romantic relationships in the past 18 months, and up to three others with whom they had had non-romantic sexual relationships. Because some of these romantic and sexual partners are also in the study (often by chance, and in the saturated settings by design), these data make it possible to construct romantic relationship and sexual partnership networks. Consequently, the risk and spread of STDs can be studied from an actual network transmission model based on empirical data; and researchers can compare sexual networks with friendship networks.

In order to protect the confidentiality of *Add Health* respondents, raw social network nomination data are not publicly available. To provide researchers with social network data arising from *Add Health*, much of our early effort on *Add Health* was directed towards developing the network data for the public use and contract data sets.

The vast majority (85 percent) of all friendship nominations and roughly 50 percent of the romantic partnership and non-romantic sexual relationships were other students in the sampled schools. Consequently, we have extensive sociometric data on friendships for the adolescents in 144 schools, and two additional waves of friendship data for the two large saturated field settings. Further, in our saturated field settings we obtained relatively complete images of romantic partnership and sexual network structures as they unfolded over time. Focusing on the in-school friendship nominations alone, we processed over 540,000 friendship nominations between 82,629 respondents in 121 schools, which provide the central focal point for social relations throughout the junior and senior high years. Despite the general sense that the adolescent friendship environment is critical for shaping adolescent health and health-risk behaviors, few people have had the opportunity to see what these large-scale networks look like at multiple levels of observation or to estimate their effects across different social contexts. *Add Health* provides such opportunities; progress along these fronts is described in more detail below.

In the course of our preliminary work with the nomination data, we constructed hundreds of variables at multiple levels of observation, from characteristics of each individual's ego-network, the structural composition of these networks and the behaviors of all friends in the sent, received, and sent and received networks, to group level (peer group), and school level networks. For each individual we have constructed numerous variables that define individual position in the school social network, including centrality, reach, maximum reach, prestige, and influence domain among others (Wasserman and Faust 1994).

For each school we have constructed detailed measures of the global network structure from density at maximum reach to centralization. In addition, for each school we have calculated in-group preference for friendships based on gender, race, and ethnicity. For the first time, multiple levels of social network data are available on the same population, thus making possible the analysis of multilevel network models across a diverse set of outcome variables (for related treatments, see Frank 1996; van Duijn et al. 1999). These publicly available constructed network variables are more fully described in *The Add Health Network Variables Codebook* (Bearman et al. 1997). The composition of each individual's peer context (at multiple levels of observation) is a key component of the network data set developed for *Add Health*.

8.4 SUMMARY OF SELECTED NETWORK FINDINGS

The wealth of network data in *Add Health* makes numerous distinct studies possible. Here we briefly summarize some of the analyses our group has completed. We focus on analyses using a range of social network data—from sexual networks to friendship networks—and highlight the diversity of dependent variables one can consider— from sexual behavior to suicidality and friendship choice.

8.4.1 The structure of adolescent sexual and romantic networks

Systematic differences in the sexual network structures that govern patterns of direct and indirect contact can have striking implications for disease transmission (Jacquez et al. 1988; Gupta and Anderson 1989; Anderson 1990; Morris 1993; Klovdahl 1995; Kretzschmar and Morris 1996; Morris 1997). Yet aside from a few studies (many of which are reported on in this volume) arising from ego-centered or snowball samples, the actual structure of sexual networks remains largely unknown. Our research identifies the structure of a complete sexual and romantic network amongst interacting adolescent residing in a mid-sized mid-western town (Bearman et al. 2003). Drawing from one of the saturated settings, we are able to describe the complete structure of all romantic and sexual relationships within an 18-month period in a single school, involving roughly 800 students.

Though the sexual network in this school is highly connected, the connectivity depends on long chains of ties, and is therefore extremely fragile. Critical to our observed network is the pronounced absence of cycles. In contrast to theoretical expectation, the observed structure of the sexual network does not appear to have a core. The absence of cycles guarantees that we are unable to observe a densely interconnected core functioning as a disease reservoir. Rather, we observe a spanning tree, characterized by the specific absence of cycles of length four (Harary 1969). A cycle of length four would be produced if, from a girl's perspective, she were to have sex with her former partner's current partner's former partner. We show that we can almost exactly replicate the structural features of the observed network, with respect to size reach, centralization, density, and number of cycles, through simulation given a prohibition against the formation of cycles of length four.

8.4.2 Peer influence on sexual debut and pregnancy risk

Most analyses of peer influence on sexual behavior concentrate solely on best friends (Billy et al. 1984; Billy and Udry 1985; Brown and Theobald 1995). Results from these studies generally show little influence. In contrast to studies of best friends, Bearman and Brückner's (Bearman and Brückner 1999) work considers network influences on sexual behavior by focusing on the structure of social relationships in which adolescents are embedded. Specifically, Bearman and Brückner consider influences that arise from social networks observed at a level more distal than best friend: the ego-network, the peer group, the leading crowd, and the school as a whole. They show that social relations have a significant influence on both sexual debut and pregnancy risk when distal network structures are considered. These influences tend to be positive, in that having a more developed social network tends to delay intercourse or reduce pregnancy risk, controlling for the risk status of individuals (Bearman and Brückner 1999). Most critical are influences that arise from the larger ego-networks in which individuals are embedded. The influence of more distal social relationships is stronger for girls than it is for boys; likewise, girls are more likely to be positively influenced than boys. This finding suggests that relationality operates differentially by gender for adolescents.

8.4.3 Social networks and adolescent suicidality

Bearman and Moody (Bearman and Moody 2004) consider the effect of social networks on suicidality. The main outcome measures are (*a*) has the adolescent seriously considered suicide in the last 12 months and (*b*) if yes, has he or she attempted suicide. They show that among adolescent males, 10.2 percent thought about suicide and 2.2 percent attempted suicide. Among females, 16 percent thought about suicide and 5 percent attempted suicide in the last year. For all adolescents, they find a strong relationship between suicidal thoughts and depression (+), experience with suicide among friends or family (+), heavy drinking (+), parental distance (+), and having a gun in the household (+). Additionally, for females we find a strong relationship between suicidality and having no friends (+), having friends who are not friends with each other (+), self-esteem (−) nonconsensual sexual relations (+), same-sex romantic attraction (+), age (−), attachment to school (−), getting into fights (+), and body-mass index (+). For males, we find playing a team sport reduces the odds of suicidal thoughts.

Females are more likely than males to attempt suicide (odds ratio 1.59). Conditional on having suicidal thoughts, there are few sex differences in the pattern of risk factors associated with attempting suicide. These analyses suggest that above and beyond the effects of depression, the social environment affects suicidality for both males and females through knowledge and exposure to suicide among friends and family. For females, suicidal thoughts are substantially increased by social isolation and dissonant local friendship patterns, nonconsensual sexual relations, and romantic attraction to other females. These social and relational factors have little impact on boys' risk of suicidal thoughts or attempts, echoing the findings we observe for sexual debut that suggest that relationality plays a more critical role for girls than it does for boys.

8.4.4 The structure of adolescent friendship networks

Moody (2002) used *Add Health* social network data to describe friendship patterns among adolescents and to test balance theory models of friendship formation and change (Moody 2002). He finds that with in-school friendship, networks tend to form clustered hierarchies embedded within a loosely connected web of students who are involved in multiple friendship groups. The friendship groups identified in these networks tend to be homogeneous with respect to many attributes and behaviors. In addition to actor similarity (Cohen 1977; Kandel 1978) and organizational opportunity factors (Feld 1981), social balance is one of the strongest predictors of friendship choice.[13] Extending traditional balance models to account for differences in transitivity from each student's point-of-view, Moody shows that a student's friendship relations are more likely to form if they increase transitivity and decrease intransitivity. Since the same pattern of relations can be transitive from one person's point of view and intransitive from another's, such actions need not lead to the static crystallized structures often hypothesized within the balance literature (Davis 1970; Davis and Leinhardt 1972). Instead, each actor's attempt to create local balance leads to new imbalances for others, which spurs further relational change.

Indeed, the school networks are not static and the observed friendship groups change as people with bridging friendships bring disconnected groups together or dissolve previous groups. In the *Add Health* data, the level of change between time points was quite high. Overall, about half of all time 2 (in-home *Wave I*) friendships are new friendship relations, with reciprocated relations at time 1 (in-school) having a much higher retention rate (between 75 and 80 percent). However, while change in particular friendships is common, large-scale status change is uncommon. Thus, popular students at time 1 tend to be popular at time 2 (mean correlation of about 0.6), with few students moving far in the popularity rankings. The greatest movement occurs among middle-ranked students, with less than 20 percent of those in the third quintile, for example, remaining in the third quintile a year later compared to over 50 percent at either tail of the distribution. Friendship relations that crossed race lines, were asymmetric, or contributed to intransitivity were all less likely to be maintained than those that fell within race, grade, or increased ego's local balance.

8.5 FUTURE DATA COLLECTION FOR *ADD HEALTH*: *SURVEY 2000*

Additional funding has been secured that will support an additional wave of *Add Health* data collection. The follow-up survey, *Survey 2000*, is planned to go into the field in January 2001.[14] At the time of our next contact, the *Add Health* sample respondents will be between 18 and 26. In addition to interviewing the full *Wave I* sample, as part of *Survey 2000* we will also interview a supplemental sample of 2000 romantic and sexual partners. Like the other waves of in-home data collection, *Survey 2000* will use the CASI format. Since we expect that many of these respondents will have

---

[13] Social balance theory (Davis 1970; Davis and Leinhardt 1972) is a theory of action stating that actors seek to avoid dissonance in their social relations. For instance, if Ann and Betty are friends, and Ann dislikes Carole, balance theory predicts that Betty will also dislike Carole. Balanced triads are transitive; unbalanced triads are intransitive.

[14] Initially, this study was scheduled to go into the field in 2000. However, project complications have delayed the anticipated start date.

experienced major changes in their lives during the past 4 years,[15] the questionnaire will make extensive use of an event history/life calendar approach to data collection. The structure of the questionnaire is designed to enhance the autobiographical memory process, and rests on identifying important events in the life course as supports for accurate dating of specific events of interest. As in previous waves of *Add Health*, *Survey 2000* contains several design elements that will facilitate the collection of network data; these design elements are discussed further below.

8.5.1 Network data in Survey 2000

Although most respondents will no longer be affiliated with local schools or other common focal institutions, we are committed to measuring network characteristics at multiple levels in *Survey 2000*. The study has been designed in order to provide accurate measures of the current local networks in which individuals are embedded, the transition dynamics governing friendship retention and loss during the transition to adulthood, baselines from which calculation of global network structures can be made, and complete images of tangible sexual networks amongst interacting young adults across diverse sociological contexts.

Specifically, the newly collected data will (*a*) enumerate current ego-networks for all respondents using multiple name generators; (*b*) describe the characteristics of respondents friends with respect to sexual behavior and risk status; (*c*) identify the current relationship between each respondent and a subset of their *Waves I* and *II* friends and sexual partners; (*d*) assess the relationships the respondents have to a random sample of individuals from their old school in order to estimate global characteristics of young adult networks from local networks; and (*e*) identify and interview both casual romantic partners and long duration partners.

8.5.2 Ego-network data in Survey 2000

Unlike the earlier waves of network data, which rested on identifying alters from a previously defined roster, in *Survey 2000* we will utilize more familiar strategies for collecting ego-centered data (similar to those used in the General Social Survey (GSS), Burt 1984, 1987). Initially, respondents will be asked to identify a set of alters with whom they share some relation r (in the GSS network module, r is "talked about important matters"). Respondents will then describe these alters with respect to standard social demographic characteristics. Finally, respondents will report on relations among their alters, thereby enabling us to calculate local ego-network density. This strategy will be used with several different relationships r, which will provide for richer and more interpretable ego-networks than does the single name generator "talked about important matters."

---

[15] We expect that roughly 20% of young adults interviewed in *Survey 2000* will be married or in marriage-like relationships, while another 25% will be in serious relationships of long duration. Roughly 25% will be in a casual dating relationship which may or may not involve sexual intercourse. Those remaining will not have a current romantic relationship.

8.5.3 *Longitudinal network data in* Survey 2000

Though social network elements are increasingly included in the design of demographic data collection projects, there is still little longitudinal network data available from important substantive contexts (for reviews, see Weesie and Flap 1990; Doreian and Stockman 1996; Suitor et al. 1997). Building from the highly clustered design of *Add Health*, *Survey 2000* offers unique opportunities to study the evolution and devolution of social networks (and their impact on social behavior) over time. The novel design exploits the friendship and romantic partnership data collected in *Waves I* and *II* of *Add Health* in order to measure changes in the composition of ego-networks as well as to derive estimates of the durability of global network structures. In *Survey 2000*, each respondent will be asked to consider their current relationship to *specific* individuals (identified by name in the CASI program) who meet the following criteria: (*a*) are in the *Survey 2000* sample; *and* (*b*) were nominated by the respondent as a friend in *Waves I* and *II*; *or* (*c*) nominated the respondent as a friend in *Waves I* or *II* but whose nomination was not reciprocated; *or* (*d*) were not in either the respondents' sent or received ego-network but were drawn from a random sample of individuals from the respondents' PSU.

For each of the selected individuals, we ask the respondent if they still know him or her, what type of relationship they are in, frequency of contact if any, date of relationship dissolution (if dissolved), and reason for dissolution. Using an event history calendar directly incorporated into the CASI interview, we will date relationship dissolution along with other salient events since last interview. Because in this section we solicit information *only* about individuals who will also be interviewed in *Survey 2000* (and from whom we will collect self-reported social demographic, behavior, and friendship network data), respondents need not describe the characteristics of these alters. The strength of this design is that for each individual, we collect data on both retained and dissolved friendship relations, while the random sample network provides the analytic leverage to estimate global features of the friendship network. We expect that we will have data on thousands of time ordered reciprocal pairs of individuals in which each partner describes the nature of his or her relationship with the other partner.

8.5.4 *Partner samples*

Beyond the ego- and longitudinal-network data collection elements, *Survey 2000* will recruit a supplemental sample of 2000 partners of *Add Health* respondents. One thousand of these partners will be randomly selected from the romantic partnerships of young adults in the core sample, while an additional one thousand partners will be recruited from the two large saturated field settings (the ethnically heterogeneous major SMSA (Standard Metropolitan Statistical Area) and the all-White Midwestern working-class community).[16] Partners will be recruited into the study using two

---

[16] Respondents will be randomly selected to provide partnership data. If they are drawn into the "provide partner" sample, they will be given protocol 1 if appropriate, otherwise they will be given protocol 2.

different protocols. The first protocol will select and then directly recruit marriage or marriage-like partners. The second protocol rests on indirect recruitment of casual partners, and is much more complex than the first protocol. Since it is nonstandard, we describe the second protocol in detail below.

The goal of the second protocol is to ensure that we will be able to match data from ego and partner without retaining individual identifiers from respondents or potential partners. To do this, we will begin with a name generator to identify individuals with whom the respondent has done things with in the past week.[17] This will yield, for each respondent, a set of names of "potential partners." Once the potential partners from all respondents have been identified, their names will be used to generate a sampling frame for the supplemental sample. We will draw a 50 percent sample of partners from this list; thus, for any individual respondent, we may attempt to recruit zero, one, or two of the individuals they have identified as a potential partner.

We will ask both the original respondent and the supplemental sample of partners to identify themselves with respect to behaviors and characteristics that are relatively rare in the population yet are likely to be known even in the early stages of a casual relationship.[18] We will also ask both the original respondent and the sample of partners to describe *their partner* with respect to the same array of characteristics.[19] From these reports we will generate pairs of vectors describing the potential partnership from two vantage points. Since egos' partners data can be compared with partners' self-report, and vice-versa, we hope that from these multiple reports we will be able to determine pairs of individuals who have a casual romantic relationship. In a pretest of this strategy, partners agreed on their partner's attributes 90 percent of the time, while the random match among unpartnered pairs of individuals was 65.2 percent. These results suggest that this design will effectively identify partnerships of low emotional intensity and short duration without violating human subject norms.

8.6 CONCLUSION

From the outset, the *Add Health* study was designed as a network study. Social networks provide a direct link between individuals and the social structure they are embedded in; for adolescents, networks of peers and friends are one of the most important social contexts, particularly with respect to health outcomes. Since most American adolescents' social worlds revolve around their school, the study draws its respondents from a carefully selected sample of schools. Since many students (and in some cases, *all* students) from sampled schools participated, *Add Health* was able to collect directed sociometric data from relatively large populations of students. Further, the use of a school-specific roster allows us to assess the characteristics of

---

[17] This name generator will be a modification of the name generator we will use to collect ego-network data.

[18] For example, body tattoos, cigarette brand, number and type of pets in the household, and birth month.   [19] We will also ask respondents to assign a "certainty score" for each item.

other members of a respondent's local, social and sexual network, without relying on respondents' reports of their partners' characteristics. Perhaps most importantly, the roster-based nomination strategy, in conjunction with the complete population coverage, allows researchers to identify the existence of structural bridges, holes, and cliques in the social and sexual networks of American adolescents. The implications of these structural characteristics of networks for both individual behavior and disease transmission have been theoretically foreshadowed for the past several decades; for the first time, we are able to evaluate them empirically.

References

Adcock, A. G., Nagy, S., and Simpson, J. A. (1991). "Selected risk factors in adolescent suicide attempts," *Adolescence*, 26: 817–28.

Anderson, J. (1990). "AIDS in Thailand," *BMJ*, 300(6722): 415–16.

Bauman, K. E. and Fisher, L. E. (1986). "Findings from longitudinal studies of adolescent smoking and drinking," *J Youth and Adolescence*, 15: 345–53.

Bearman, P. (1991). "The social structure of suicide," *Sociol Forum*, 6(3): 501–24.

—— and Brückner, H. (1999). *Power in Numbers: Peer Effects on Adolescent Girls' Sexual Debut and Pregnancy*. Washington DC: National Campaign to Prevent Teen Pregnancy.

—— Moody, J., and Stovel, K. (1997). *The Add Health Network Variable Codebook*. University of North Carolina at Chapel Hill.

—————— (2004). "Chains of Affection: The structure of adolescent romantic and sexual networks." *American Journal of Sociology* (in press).

—— and Moody, J. (2004). "Adolescent suicidality," *Am J Public Health* (in press).

Bearman, P. S., Jones, J., and Udry, J. R. (1996). *Connections Count: The Add Health Design*. www.cpc.unc.edu/projects/addhealth/design.html.

Billy, J. and Udry, J. R. (1985). "The influence of male and female best friends on adolescent sexual behavior," *Adolescence*, 20: 21–32.

Billy, J. O. G., Rodgers, J. L., and Udry, J. R. (1984). "Adolescent Sexual Behavior and Friendship Choice," *Social Forces*, 62(3): 753–78.

Brown, B. B. and Theobald, W. (1995). "How Peers Matter: A Research Synthesis of Peer Influences on Adolescent Pregnancy." In *Peer Potential: Making the Most of How Teens Influence Each Other*. Washington DC: The National Campaign to Prevent Teen Pregnancy.

Burt, R. S. (1984). "Network items and the general social survey," *Soc Net*, 6: 293–339.

—— (1987). "Social contagion and innovation: Cohesion versus structural equivalence," *American Journal of Sociology*, 92: 1287–335.

Cohen, J. M. (1977). "Sources of peer group homogeneity," *Sociol Educ*, 50: 227–41.

Davis, J. A. (1970). "Clustering and hierarchy in interpersonal relations: Testing two graph theoretical models on 742 sociomatrices," *Am Sociol Rev*, 35: 843–51.

—— and Leinhardt, S. (1972). *The Structure of Positive Relations in Small Groups*. Boston, MA: Houghton Mifflin.

Doreian, P. and Stockman, F. (1996). *Evolution of Social Networks*. New York, NY: Gordon and Breach.

Feld, S. (1981). "The focused organization of social ties," *Am J Sociol*, 86: 1015–35.

Frank, K. A. (1996). "Mapping interactions within and between cohesive subgroups," *Soc Net*, 18: 93–119.

Gupta, S. and Anderson, R. (1989). "Networks of sexual contacts: Implications for the pattern of spread of HIV," *AIDS*, 3: 807–17.

Harary, F. (1969). *Graph Theory. Reading*. Massachusetts: Addison-Wesley.

Hayes, C. D. E. (1987). *Risking the Future: Adolescent Sexuality, Pregnancy, and Childbearing*. Washington DC: National Academy Press.

Jacquez, J., Simon, C., Koopman, J. et al. (1988). "Modeling and analyzing HIV transmission: The effect of contact patterns," *Math Biosc*, 92: 119–99.

Jeanneret, O. (1992). "A tentative epidemiologic approach to suicide prevention in adolescence," *J Adolescent Health*, 13: 409–14.

Kandel, D. B. (1978). "Convergences in prospective longitudinal surveys of drug use in normal populations." In D. B. Kandel (ed.) *Longitudinal Research on Drug Use: Empirical Findings and Methodological Issues*. New York, NY: John Wiley and Sons.

Klovdahl, A. S. (1995). "Social networks: Special edition on social networks and infectious disease," *HIV/AIDS*, 17: Amsterdam, Netherlands: Elsevier Science BV.

Kretzschmar, M. and Morris, M. (1996). "Measures of concurrency in networks and the spread of infectious disease," *Math Biosc*, 133: 165–95.

Laumann, E., Gagnon, J., Michael, R. T. et al. (1994). *The Social Organization of Sexuality: Sexual Practices in the United States*. Chicago, IL: The University of Chicago Press.

Moody, J. (2002). "Race, school integration, and friendship in America," *Am J Sociol*, 107: 679–716.

Morris, M. (1993). "Epidemiology and social networks: Modeling structured diffusion," *Soc Meth Res*, 22(1): 99–126.

—— (1997). "Sexual networks and HIV," *AIDS*, 11(Suppl A): S209–16.

Resnick, M. D., Bearman, P., Blum, R. W. et al. (1997). "Protecting adolescents from harm: Findings from the national longitudinal study on adolescent health," *J Am Med Assoc*, 9(10): 932–43.

Smith, K. and Crawford, S. (1986). "Suicidal behavior among 'Normal' high school students," *Suicide and Life Threatening Behavior*, 16: 313–25.

Suitor, J. J., Wellman, B., and Morgan, D. L. (1997). "It's About Time: How, Why and When Networks Change," *Soc Net*, 19(1): 1–7.

Thompson, S. (1995). *Going All the Way. Teenage Girls' Tales of Sex, Romance, and Pregnancy*. New York, NY: Hill and Wang.

Turner, C., Ku, L., Rogers, S. M. et al. (1998). "Adolescent sexual behavior, drug use, and violence: Increased reporting with computer survey technology," *Science*, May(280): 5365.

van Duijn, M. A. J., van Busschbach, J. T., and Snijders, T. A. B. (1999). "Multilevel analysis of personal networks as dependent variables," *Soc Net*, 21: 187–209.

Wasserman, S. and Faust, K. (1994). *Social Network Analysis: Methods and Applications*. Cambridge: Cambridge University Press.

Weesie, J. and Flap, H. (1990). *Social Networks Through Time*. Utrecht, Netherlands: ISOR.

Glossary

This glossary is not meant to be exhaustive list of network terminology. The best source for this is Wasserman and Faust (1994). The terms listed here are drawn from the chapters of this volume.

- Actor—A node in a network, typically a person, but can be a larger unit such as an organization or a state. The unit for which relational data are measured.
- Adjacent—Two nodes are adjacent if they are connected by some relational measure or, in a graphical representation of a network, by a line. Two relations are adjacent if they share a node.
- Adjacency matrix—A matrix in which the rows and columns represent nodes in the network and the cell values represent the relational links between them. Typically the cell values are {0, 1}, for presence or absence of a relation, but valued entries are also possible to represent intensity, duration, positive/negative affect, and other nonbinary aspects of relations.
- Alter—A partner who is nominated by a sampled respondent in response to a name generator.
- Assortative mixing—A pattern of relations among nodes in which ties among similar nodes are more likely than ties among non-similar nodes. The term comes from "assortative mating" in the population genetics literature.
- Balance Theory—An approach to network analysis that focuses on the systematic patterns of positive and negative affect among triads. For example, my friend's enemy is my enemy.
- Betweenness—A measure of centrality based on the number of times a node lies on the shortest path between each connected dyad in the network.
- Bonacich power—A measure of the prestige of a node in a network based on the prestige of the other actors to which the node is connected.
- Bridge—A node (or group of nodes) that connects two otherwise disconnected subgroups of the overall network. Bisexuals, for example, bridge between homosexual men and heterosexual women.
- Centrality—The extent to which the node is in the middle of a network, and *centralization* is a measure of the extent to which an entire network is concentrated on a common core. Many different measures have been proposed, including *degree, betweenness,* and *information* centrality.
- Clique—A subset of a network in which the actors are more densely tied to one another than to other members of the network. Definitions range from the maximally dense (all possible ties are active) to less dense "*k-cliques*," where at least *k* ties exist between every actor in the clique and other actors in the clique.
- Closeness—A measure of the typical path length between each node and every other node in the network. The inverse of the distance of each actor to every other actor in the network.

Glossary

- Cluster sampling—A sampling strategy in which respondents are sampled from clusters, or larger groupings of the population.
- Complete network data—A network data set that contains information on all of the persons in a defined group, and all of the links among them (also called sociometric data).
- Component—A subset of nodes in a network among which there is a direct or indirect path between all pairs of actors and no paths between an actor in the subset and an actor not in the subset.
- Component size—the number of nodes in a component.
- Concurrency—Relations that overlap in time. Typically used in the context of sexual relations to refer to partnerships that are not serially monogamous.
- Contact matrix—An adjacency matrix where the rows and columns are collapsed into subgroups of actors who share an attribute. The cell entries represent the number of relations between the row group and the column group. Also called a "*mixing matrix.*"
- Core—This term has a number of different field-specific definitions (from social network analysis and epidemiology). In mathematical epidemiology, the technical definition is a subgroup in a population in which the reproductive rate of the infection (R_0) is above 1, so that the epidemic can persist in that subgroup, even if the R_0 for the entire population is below 1. In network analysis, it refers to the central dense component in a network that also has a "periphery." The common aspect to both definitions is the centralized, somewhat separate, and relatively more densely connected part of a network.
- Cycle—A walk that begins and ends at the same node and involves at least three distinct nodes (see *walk*).
- Degree—The number of alters adjacent to a node or, equivalently, the number of relational ties of a node. A distinction can be made between indegree and outdegree if the relation is directed.
- Digraph—A graph with directed ties.
- Directed ties—Relations that are sent from one node and received by another node and may be unreciprocated. Friendship is an example of a directed tie, "sibling" is an example of an undirected tie.
- Disassortative mixing—Relations among nodes classified as being dissimilar on some attribute (see *assortative mixing*).
- Distance—The length of the shortest path between two nodes (see *closeness*).
- Dyad—A pair of nodes in a network, sometimes used to refer only to pairs that have a relation.
- Egocentric network data—A network data set created by sampling a set of focal actors (or egos), asking them to nominate their partners (alters), and asking them to report on the ties between their alters. See also *local* network data.
- Endogenous variable—A variable whose value is determined by the status of the other variables within the same system.
- k-plex—A clique of size n allowing nodes to be members of the clique so long as they are adjacent to at least n-k members of the clique (see clique).

- Kappa—A measure of concurrency that is based on the mean degree of the line graph.
- Kish Table—A table used to randomly select one person from a household when more than one member is eligible for participation (based on a method developed by Leslie Kish).
- Incidence—The rate at which new cases of a disease occur in a population, measured as the number of new cases divided by the number in the population at risk over a specified time period.
- Isolate—A node (person) with no partners.
- KRACKPLOT—A computer program for network visualization.
- Link sampling—(see "*snowball sample*").
- Local network data—Network data derived from a survey of respondents and information they provide on their partners, in which the partners are neither traced nor enrolled in the study. See also *egocentric* network data.
- Name generator—The questions in a network survey that are used to elicit the names of a respondent's partners.
- Nomination—A partner reported by a sampled respondent.
- Partial network data—A social network data set consisting of respondents and ties from a chain-link (or snowball) sampling strategy. This definition comprises a wide range of different designs, distinguished by the number of "generations" or "waves" of alters enrolled, and the number of alters sampled at each generation.
- Path—A sequence of adjacent nodes in which each intervening node is visited only once (see "*walk*").
- "Patient Zero"—The first HIV+ case in the United States, and the start of the chain of HIV transmission.
- Pearson's correlation coefficient—A measure of the degree of linear relationship between two variables.
- Periphery—Nodes on the margin of a network or network component.
- Prestige—A measure of status, often represented by the number of ties an actor receives in a directed network.
- Prevalence—The proportion of the population with an attribute (in epidemiology, typically an infection) at a certain time, measured as the number of cases divided by the population at risk.
- Propinquity—Closeness in relationship or character.
- Reachability—A binary measure of whether there is a path between two nodes.
- Relative risk—The probability of an event in a target group divided by the probability of the event in a control group.
- Seed—The initial sampled respondents in a snowball (chain-referral) sampling design.
- Sociogram—The graphical representation of a social network.
- Sociometric data—A social network data set consisting of a bounded group of persons and the measured relations among them (see complete network data).
- Sociomatrix—(see adjacency matrix).

- Snowball sample—An adaptive sampling strategy that uses the nominations of current respondents to identify and enroll subsequent respondents. The process continues until a designated stopping point. Also called a *link-tracing* or *chain-referral* design.
- Subgroup—A subset of individuals in a population who share an attribute.
- "Type III" transmission—A pattern of HIV transmission whereby the disease is initially spread mostly through international travel and infected blood supplies.
- Walk—A sequence of adjacent nodes.

Reference

Wasserman, S. and Faust, K. (1994). *Social Network Analysis: Methods and Applications.* Cambridge University Press: Cambridge.

Publications from Data Sets Reviewed in This Volume

CHAPTER 1

Binson, D., Michaels, S. et al. (1995). "Prevalence and social distribution of men who have sex with men—United-States and its urban centers," *J Sex Res*, 32(3): 245–54.

Bogaert, A. F., Friesen, C. et al. (2002). "Age of puberty and sexual orientation in a national probability sample," *Arch Sex Behav*, 31(1): 73–81.

Brackbill, R. M., Sternberg, M. R. et al. (1999). "Where do people go for treatment of sexually transmitted diseases?" *Fam Plann Perspect*, 31(1): 10–15.

Browning, C. R. (2002a). "The span of collective efficacy: Extending social disorganization theory to partner violence," *J Marriage and the Fam*, 64(4): 833–50.

——(2002b). "Trauma or transition: A life-course perspective on the link between childhood sexual experiences and men's adult well-being," *Soc Sci Res*, 31(4): 473–510.

—— and Laumann, E. O. (1997). "Sexual contact between children and adults: A life course perspective," *Am Sociol Rev*, 62(4): 540–60.

Catania, J. A., Canchola, J. et al. (1996). "They said it couldn't be done—The National Health and Social Life Survey—Response," *Public Opin Quart*, 60(4): 620–7.

Couper, M. P. and Stinson, L. L. (1999). "Completion of self-administered questionnaires in a sex survey," *J Sex Res*, 36(4): 321–30.

Curtis, R. L., Leung, P. et al. (2001). "Outcomes of child sexual contacts: Patterns of incarcerations from a national sample," *Child Abuse Negl*, 25(5): 719–36.

Feinleib, J. A. and Michael, R. T. (1998). "Reported changes in sexual behavior in response to AIDS in the United States," *Prev Med*, 27(3): 400–11.

Hyde, J. S., DeLamater, J. D. et al. (2001). "Sexuality and the dual-earner couple, part II: Beyond the baby years," *J Sex Res*, 38(1): 10–23.

Ku, L., Sonenstein, F. L. et al. (1997). "The promise of integrated representative surveys about sexually transmitted diseases and behavior," *Sex Transm Dis*, 24(5): 299–309.

Laumann, E. O., Masi, C. M. et al. (1997). "Circumcision in the United States—Prevalence, prophylactic effects, and sexual practice," *JAMA-J Am Med Assoc*, 277(13): 1052–7.

—— Paik, A. et al. (1999a). "Lecture 6—The epidemiology of erectile dysfunction: Results from the National Health and Social Life Survey," *Int J Impot Res*, 11: S60–4.

—— ——(1999b). "Sexual dysfunction in the United States—Prevalence and predictors," *JAMA-J Am Med Assoc*, 281(6): 537–44.

—— and Youm, Y. (1999). "Racial/ethnic group differences in the prevalence of sexually transmitted diseases in the United States: A network explanation," *Sex Transm Dis*, 26(5): 250–61.

Liu, C. (2000). "A theory of marital sexual life," *J Marriage and the Fam*, 62(2): 363–74.

——(2003). "Does quality of marital sex decline with duration?" *Arch Sex Behav*, 32(1): 55–60.

Miller, P. V. (1995). "The polls–A review—they said it couldn't be done—the national-health and social-life survey," *Pub Opin Quart*, 59(3): 404–19.

——(1996). "They said it couldn't be done: The national health and social life survey—reply," *Pub Opin Quart*, 60(4): 628–33.

Rosal, M. C., Ockene, I. S. et al. (1997). "A longitudinal study of students' depression at one medical school," *Acad Med*, 72(6): 542–6.

Yancey, G. (2003). "A preliminary examination of differential sexual attitudes among individuals involved in interracial relationships: Testing 'Jungle Fever'," *Soc Sci J*, 40(1): 153–7.

Youm, Y. and Laumann, E. O. (2002). "Social network effects on the transmission of sexually transmitted diseases," *Sex Transm Dis*, 29(11): 689–97.

see also: http://www.icpsr.umich.edu/cgi-bin/CITATIONS/search.prl?study=6647&method= study&path=ICPSR

CHAPTER 2

Morris, M. (1997). "Sexual networks and HIV," *AIDS*, 11: S209–16.

——and Kretzschmar, M. (1997). "Concurrent partnerships and the spread of HIV," *AIDS*, 11(5): 641–8.

————(2000). "A micro-simulation study of the effect of concurrent partnerships on HIV spread in Uganda," *Math Pop Stud*, 8(2): 109–33.

——and O'Gorman, J. (2000). "The impact of measurement error on survey estimates of concurrency," *Math Pop Stud*, 8(3): 231–49.

——Podhisita, C. et al. (1996). "Bridge populations in the spread of HIV/AIDS in Thailand," *AIDS*, 10(11): 1265–71.

——Pramualratana, A. et al. (1995). "The relational determinants of condom use with commercial sex partners in Thailand," *AIDS*, 9(5): 507–15.

——Wawer, M. J. et al. (2000). "Condom acceptance is higher among travelers in Uganda," *AIDS*, 14(6): 733–41.

CHAPTER 3

Auvert, B., Buve, A. et al. (2001a). "Ecological and individual level analysis of risk factors for HIV infection in four urban populations in sub-Saharan Africa with different levels of HIV infection," *AIDS*, 15: S15–30.

————(2001b). "Male circumcision and HIV infection in four cities in sub-Saharan Africa," *AIDS*, 15: S31–40.

Buve, A. (2002). "HIV epidemics in Africa: What explains the variations in HIV prevalence?" *Iubmb Life*, 53(4–5): 193–5.

——Carael, M. et al. (2001a). "Multicentre study on factors determining differences in rate of spread of HIV in sub-Saharan Africa: Methods and prevalence of HIV infection," *AIDS*, 15: S5–14.

————(2001b). "The multicentre study on factors determining the differential spread of HIV in four African cities: Summary and conclusions," *AIDS*, 15: S127–31.

——Lagarde, E. et al. (2001). "Interpreting sexual behaviour data: Validity issues in the multi-centre study on factors determining the differential spread of HIV in four African cities," *AIDS*, 15: S117–26.

——Weiss, H. A. et al. (2001a). "The epidemiology of gonorrhoea, chlamydial infection and syphilis in four African cities," *AIDS*, 15: S79–88.

————(2001b). "The epidemiology of trichomoniasis in women in four African cities," *AIDS*, 15: S89–96.

Ferry, B., Carael, M. et al. (2001). "Comparison of key parameters of sexual behaviour in four African urban populations with different levels of HIV infection," *AIDS*, 15: S41–50.

Lagarde, E., Auvert, B. et al. (2001*a*). "Concurrent sexual partnerships and HIV prevalence in five urban communities of sub-Saharan Africa," *AIDS*, 15(7): 877–84.

—— —— (2001*b*). "Condom use and its associations with HIV/sexually transmitted diseases in four urban communities of sub-Saharan Africa," *AIDS*, 15: S71–8.

—— Carael, M. et al. (2001). "Educational level is associated with condom use within non-spousal partnerships in four cities of sub-Saharan Africa," *AIDS*, 15(11): 1399–408.

Morison, L., Buve, A. et al. (2001). "HIV-1 subtypes and the HIV epidemics in four cities in sub-Saharan Africa," *AIDS*, 15: S109–16.

—— Weiss, H. A. et al. (2001). "Commercial sex and the spread of HIV in four cities in sub-Saharan Africa," *AIDS*, 15: S61–9.

Weiss, H. A., Buve, A. et al. (2001). "The epidemiology of HSV-2 infection and its association with HIV infection in four urban African populations," *AIDS*, 15: S97–108.

CHAPTER 4

Jolly, A. M., Muth, S. Q. et al. (2001). "Sexual networks and sexually transmitted infections: A tale of two cities," *J Urban Health*, 78(3): 433–45.

Klovdahl, A. S., Potterat, J. J. et al. (1994). "Social networks and infectious-disease—the Colorado-Springs study," *Soc Sci Med*, 38(1): 79–88.

Potterat, J. J., Muth, S. Q. et al. (2002). "Sexual network structure as an indicator of epidemic phase," *Sex Transm Infect*, 78: I152–8.

—— Phillips-Plummer, L. et al. (2002). "Risk network structure in the early epidemic phase of HIV transmission in Colorado Springs," *Sex Transm Infect*, 78: I159–63.

—— Woodhouse, D. E. et al. (1993). "Aids in Colorado-Springs—is there an epidemic," *AIDS*, 7(11): 1517–21.

—— Zimmerman-Rogers, H. et al. (1999). "Chlamydia transmission: Concurrency, reproduction number, and the epidemic trajectory," *Amer J Epidemiol*, 150(12): 1331–9.

Rothenberg, R. B., Potterat, J. J. et al. (1995). "Choosing a centrality measure—epidemiologic correlates in the Colorado-Springs study of social networks," *Soc Nets*, 17(3–4): 273–97.

—— —— (1998). "Social network dynamics and HIV transmission," *AIDS*, 12(12): 1529–36.

Woodhouse, D. E., Rothenberg, R. B. et al. (1994). "Mapping a social network of heterosexuals at high-risk for HIV-infection," *AIDS*, 8(9): 1331–6.

CHAPTER 5

Baldwin, J. A., Trotter, R. T. et al. (1999). "HIV/AIDS risks among native American drug users: Key findings from focus group interviews and implications for intervention strategies," *AIDS Educ Prev*, 11(4): 279–92.

Rothenberg, R., Baldwin, J. et al. (2001). "The risk environment for HIV transmission: Results from the Atlanta and Flagstaff network studies," *J Urban Health—Bull NY Acad Med*, 78(3): 419–32.

—— Kimbrough, L. et al. (2000). "Social network methods for endemic foci of syphilis—a pilot project," *Sex Transm Dis*, 27(1): 12–18.

Rothenberg, R. B., Long, D. M. et al. (2000). "The Atlanta urban networks study: A blueprint for endemic transmission," *AIDS*, 14(14): 2191–200.

CHAPTER 6

Aral, S. O., Hughes, J. P. et al. (1999). "Sexual mixing patterns in the spread of gonococcal and chlamydial infections," *Am J Public Health*, 89(6): 825–33.

Foxman, B., Aral, S. O. et al. (1998). "Heterosexual repertoire is associated with same-sex experience," *Sex Transm Dis*, 25(5): 232–6.

Garnett, G. P., Hughes, J. P. et al. (1996). "Sexual mixing patterns of patients attending sexually transmitted diseases clinics," *Sex Transm Dis*, 23(3): 248–57.

Gorbach, P. M., Aral, S. O. et al. (2000). "Notify or not to notify—STD patients' perspectives of partner notification in Seattle," *Sex Transm Dis*, 27(4): 193–200.

——— Stoner, B. P. et al. (2002). " 'It takes a village'—understanding concurrent sexual partnerships in Seattle, Washington," *Sex Transm Dis*, 29(8): 453–62.

Manhart, L. E., Aral, S. O. et al. (2002). "Sex partner concurrency—Measurement, prevalence, and correlates among urban 18–39-year-olds," *Sex Transm Dis*, 29(3): 133–43.

Stoner, B. P., Whittington, W. L. et al. (2000). "Comparative epidemiology of heterosexual gonococcal and chlamydial networks—Implications for transmission patterns," *Sex Transm Dis*, 27(4): 215–23.

CHAPTER 7

Alva, Soumya and Entwisle, Barbara (2002). "Employment transitions in an era of change in Thailand," *Journal of Southeast Asian Studies*, 40(3): 303–26.

Chamratrithirong, Aphichat and Sethaput, Chanya (eds.) (1997). *Fieldwork Experiences Related to the Longitudinal Study of the Demographic Responses to a Changing Environment in Nang Rong, 1994*. Mahidol University: Institute for Population and Social Research.

1. Chanya Sethaput. Introduction.
2. Chanya Sethaput and Aphichat Chamratrithirong. "Fieldwork design."
3. Thirapong Santiphop. "Data collection of the community profile."
4. Aree Jampaklay. "Data collection of the old and new households."
5. Kanchana Tangchonlatip. "Migrant follow-up study."
6. Aphichat Chamratrithirong. Summary and Conclusion.

Curran, Sara R., Chung, Chang, Cadge, Wendy, and Varangrat, Anchalee (2002). "Boys' and girls' changing educational opportunities in Thailand: The effects of siblings, migration, and village remoteness." Office of Population Research Working Paper No. 2002–5. Princeton, NJ: Princeton University.

———, ———, ———, and ——— (forthcoming) "Boys' and girls' changing educational opportunities in Thailand: The effects of siblings, migration, and village remoteness." *Review of Sociology of Education*.

———, Entwisle, B., Jampaklay, A. (2000). "Postnuptial residence as an expression of social change in Nang Rong, Thailand." Office of Population Research Working Paper No. 2000–2. Princeton, NJ: Princeton University.

———, Garip, Filiz, Chung, Chang, and Tangchonlatip, Kanchana (2003). "Gendered migrant social capital: Evidence from Thailand," Center for Migration and Development Working Paper #03-12, Office of Population Research. Princeton, NJ: Princeton University.

Entwisle, B., Rindfuss, R. R., Guilkey, D. K., Chamratrithirong, A., Curran, S. R., and Sawangdee, Y. (1993). "Social networks and contraceptive choice in Thailand: Lessons learned from a focus group study in Nang Rong district." In Bencha Yoddumnern-Attig and Associates (eds.), *Qualitative Methods for Population and Health Research*. Salaya, Thailand: Institute for Population and Social Research. Mahidol University.

——, ——, ——, ——, ——, and —— (1996). "Community and contraceptive choice in rural Thailand: A case study of Nang Rong," *Demography* 33(1): 1–11.

——, ——, Walsh, S. J., Evans, T. P., and Curran, S. R. (1997). "Geographic information systems, spatial network analysis, and contraceptive choice," *Demography* 34: 171–87.

——, Walsh, S. J., Rindfuss, R. R., and Chamratrithirong, A. (1998). "Landuse/landcover and population dynamics, Nang Rong, Thailand." In D. Liverman, E. F. Moran, R. R. Rindfuss, and P. C. Stern (eds.), *People and Pixels: Using Remotely Sensed Data in Social Science Research*. National Academy Press, National Academy of Sciences, Committee on the Human Dimensions of Global Change, Washington, DC, pp. 121–44.

Evans, T. P., Walsh, S. J., Entwisle, B., and Rindfuss, R. R. (1995). "Testing model parameters of transportation Network analyses in rural Thailand." In Proceedings, GIS/LIS '95, vol. I. Bethesda, MD: American Society for Photogrammetry and Remote Sensing: American Congress on Surveying and Mapping, pp. 302–11.

Faust, K., Entwisle, B., Rindfuss, R. R., Walsh, S. J., and Sawangdee, Y. (1999). "Spatial arrangements of social and economic networks among villages in Nang Rong district, Thailand," *Social Networks*, 21(4): 311–37.

Godley, J. (2001). "Kinship networks and contraceptive choice in Nang Rong, Thailand," *International Family Planning Perspectives*, pp. 4–10, 41.

Institute for Population and Social Research (IPSR) (1984). "A Demographic, Socioeconomic, and Health Profile of a Rural Community in Nang Rong," Bangkok, Thailand: Institute for Population and Social Research, Mahidol University.

Rindfuss, R. R., Entwisle, B., Walsh, S. J., Prasakurt, P., Sawangdee, Y., Crawford, T. W., and Reade, J. (2002). "Continuous and discrete: Where they have met in Nang Rong, Thailand." In S. J. Walsh and K. A. Crews-Meyer (eds.), *Remote Sensing and GIS Applications for Linking People, Place, and Policy*. Norwell, MA: Kluwer Academic Publishers, pp. 7–37.

——, Guilkey, D. K., Entwisle, B., Chamratrithirong, A., and Sawangdee, Y. (1996). "The family building life course and contraceptive use: Nang Rong, Thailand," *Population Research and Policy Review* 15: 341–68.

——, Prasartkul, P., Walsh, S. J., Entwisle, B., Sawangdee, Y., Vogler, J. B. (2003). "Household-parcel linkages in Nang Rong, Thailand: Challenges of large samples." In Jefferson Fox, Ronald R. Rindfuss, Stephen J. Walsh, and Vinod Mishra, (eds.), *People and the Environment: Approaches for Linking Household and Community Surveys to Remote Sensing and GIS*. Boston, MA: Kluwer Academic Publishers, pp. 131–72.

VanWey, Leah K. (2003). "Land ownership as a determinant of temporary migration in Nang Rong, Thailand," *European Journal of Population*, 19: 121–45.

Walsh, S. J. (1999). "Deforestation and agricultural extensification in northeast Thailand: A remote sensing and GIS study of landscape structure and scale." Proceedings, Applied Geography Conference, 22: 223–32.

——, Crawford, T. W., Welsh, W. F., and Crews-Meyer, K. A. (2001). "A multiscale analysis of LULC and NDVI variation in Nang Rong district, Northeast Thailand," *Agriculture Ecosystems and Environment*, 85(1–3): 47–64.

——, Crews-Meyer, K. A., Crawford, T. W., and Welsh, W. F. (2001). "Population and environment interactions: Spatial considerations in landscape characterization and modeling." In R. McMaster and E. Sheppard (eds.), *Scale and Geographic Inquiry: Nature, Society, and Method*. Blackwell Publishers.

230 *Publications from data sets reviewed in this volume*

Walsh, S. J., Crews-Meyer, K. A., Crawford, T. W., Welsh, W. F., Entwisle, B., and Rindfuss, R. R. (2001). "Patterns of change in LULC and plant biomass: Separating intra- and inter-annual signals in monsoon-driven northeast Thailand." In A. C. Millington, S. J. Walsh, and P. E. Osborne (eds.), *Remote Sensing and GIS Applications in Biogeography and Ecology*. Kluwer Academic Publishers: Boston, pp. 91–108.

——, ——, and Messina, J. P. (2000). "Landscape variation in frontier environments: The case of agricultural extensification in Ecuador and Thailand." 4th International Conference on Integrating GIS and Environmental Modeling, Banff, Canada.

——, Entwisle, B., and Rindfuss, R. R. (1998). "Population-environment interactions in Thailand: Landscape characterization through remote sensing, GIS and population surveys." In S. Morain (ed.), *GIS Solutions in Natural Resource Management*. Albuquerque, NM: Onward Press, pp. 251–65.

——, ——, and —— (1999). "Landscape characterization through remote sensing, GIS and population surveys." In S. Morain (ed.), *GIS Solutions in Natural Resource Management: Balancing The Technical-Political Equation*. Santa Fe: OnWord Press First Edition, pp. 251–65.

——, Evans, T. P., Welsh, W. F., Entwisle, B., and Rindfuss, R. R. (1999). "scale-dependent relationships between population and environment in northeastern Thailand," *Photogrammetric Engineering & Remote Sensing*, 65(1): 97–105.

——, ——, ——, Rindfuss, R. R., and Entwisle, B. (1998). "Population and environmental characteristics associated with village boundaries and landuse/landcover patterns in Nang Rong district, Thailand." Proceedings of Pecora 13, Symposium on Human Interactions with the Environment: Perspectives from Space. Bethesda, MD: American Society for Photogrammetry and Remote Sensing.

CHAPTER 8

Alexander, C., Piazza, M. et al. (2001). "Peers, schools, and adolescent cigarette smoking," *J Adolescent Health*, 29(1): 22–30.

Bankston, C. L. and Zhou, M. (2002). "Social capital as process: The meanings and problems of a theoretical metaphor," *Sociol Inquiry*, 72(2): 285–317.

Bearman, P. S. (2002). "Opposite-sex twins and adolescent same-sex attraction," *Am J Sociol*, 107(5): 1179–205.

—— and Bruckner, H. (2001). "Promising the future: Virginity pledges and first intercourse," *Am J Sociol*, 106(4): 859–912.

Cleveland, H. H. and Wiebe, R. P. (2003). "The moderation of adolescent-to-peer similarity in tobacco and alcohol use by school levels of substance use," *Child Develop*, 74(1): 279–91.

Crosnoe, R. and Elder, G. H. (2002). "Adolescent twins and emotional distress: The interrelated influence of nonshared environment and social structure," *Child Develop*, 73(6): 1761–74.

Ford, K., Sohn, W. et al. (2001). "Characteristics of adolescents' sexual partners and their association with use of condoms and other contraceptive methods," *Fam Plann Perspect*, 33(3): 100–5.

Halpern, C. T., Oslak, S. G. et al. (2001). "Partner violence among adolescents in opposite-sex romantic relationships: Findings from the National Longitudinal Study of Adolescent Health," *Am J Public Health*, 91(10): 1679–85.

Haynie, D. L. (2001). "Delinquent peers revisited: Does network structure matter?" *Am J Sociol*, 106(4): 1013–57.

—— (2002). "Friendship networks and delinquency: The relative nature of peer delinquency," *J Quantitative Criminol*, 18(2): 99–134.

Joyner, K. and Kao, G. (2000). "School racial composition and adolescent racial homophily," *Soc Sci Quart*, 81(3): 810–25.

Kaestle, C. E., Morisky, D. E. et al. (2002). "Sexual intercourse and the age difference between adolescent females and their romantic partners," *Perspect Sexual Reproduct Health*, 34(6): 304–9.

Kelley, S. S., Borawski, E. A. et al. (2003). "The role of sequential and concurrent sexual relationships in the risk of sexually transmitted diseases among adolescents," *J Adolescent Health*, 32(4): 296–305.

Moody, J. (2001a). "Peer influence groups: Identifying dense clusters in large networks," *Soc Nets*, 23(4): 261–83.

—— (2001b). "Race, school integration, and friendship segregation in America," *Am J Sociol*, 107(3): 679–716.

—— (2002). "The importance of relationship timing for diffusion," *Soc Forces*, 81(1): 25–56.

Russell, S. T., Franz, B. T. et al. (2001). "Same-sex romantic attraction and experiences of violence in adolescence," *Am J Public Health*, 91(6): 903–6.

Santelli, J. S., Lindberg, L. D. et al. (2000). "Adolescent sexual behavior: Estimates and trends from four nationally representative surveys," *Fam Plann Perspect*, 32(4): 156–65.

Index

Lightning Source UK Ltd.
Milton Keynes UK
UKHW010647130223
416869UK00004B/337